THE JOHNS HOPKINS GUIDE *TO*
PSYCHOLOGICAL FIRST AID

GEORGE S. EVERLY, JR. & JEFFREY M. LATING

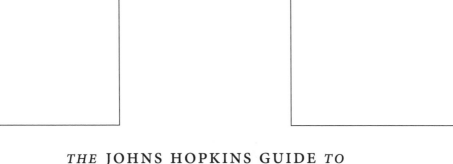

THE JOHNS HOPKINS GUIDE *TO*

PSYCHOLOGICAL FIRST AID

2ND EDITION

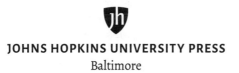

JOHNS HOPKINS UNIVERSITY PRESS
Baltimore

© 2022 Johns Hopkins University Press
All rights reserved. Published 2022
Printed in the United States of America on acid-free paper

2 4 6 8 9 7 5 3 1

Johns Hopkins University Press
2715 North Charles Street
Baltimore, Maryland 21218-4363
www.press.jhu.edu

Library of Congress Cataloging-in-Publication Data

Names: Everly, George S., Jr., 1950– author. | Lating, Jeffrey M., author.
Title: The Johns Hopkins guide to psychological first aid / George S. Everly, Jr.,
  Jeffrey M. Lating.
Description: Second edition. | Baltimore : Johns Hopkins University Press, 2022. |
  Includes bibliographical references and index.
Identifiers: LCCN 2021048348 | ISBN 9781421443997 (paperback) |
  ISBN 9781421444000 (ebook)
Subjects: LCSH: Crisis intervention (Mental health services) | Psychiatric
  emergencies. | Stress (Psychology)—Prevention.
Classification: LCC RC480.6 .E91145 2022 | DDC 616.89/025—dc23/eng/20211012
LC record available at https://lccn.loc.gov/2021048348

A catalog record for this book is available from the British Library.

Special discounts are available for bulk purchases of this book.
For more information, please contact Special Sales at
specialsales@jh.edu.

To the pioneers who gave birth to the field of disaster mental health—what an amazing journey it has been. We didn't always get it right at first, but we kept trying until we did. Consistent with that theme, we craft this second edition with the intention of continuing the journey of improvement and innovation.

To my father, George S. Everly, Sr. And to Patricia Copps Everly and our mutual renaissance! Thank you! And to George S. Everly IV and to Henry Paul Everly, may the world you inherit be a kinder and more peaceful place.

GSE

To all those who have taught me so much about the field of disaster mental health. It is a privilege to be able to share what I have learned.

And to Austin and Jenna, who remain the source of my greatest joy.

JML

CONTENTS

SIX   126
A—Assessment | *Listening to the Story*

SEVEN   141
P—Psychological Triage | *Prioritization*

EIGHT   152
I—Intervention | *Tactics to Stabilize and Mitigate Acute Distress*

How Did We Get Here?

THE IMPORTANCE OF PROVIDING SUPPORT to someone in emergent distress is self-evident. Whether it's responding to the attacks of September 11, 2001, Hurricane Katrina in 2005, the terrorist attacks in Paris in 2015 and Brussels in 2016, or responding to the emotional consequences of a devastating house fire or medical crisis, there is most commonly a compelling desire to help those in distress. The years 2020–22 contain events that will define a generation: COVID-19, which arose from Wuhan, China, and the vitriolic political upheaval that arose around a presidential election, culminating not only in the election itself but in a riot at the Capitol of the United States on January 6, 2021. What may be less evident is *how* to provide assistance, especially when a person is in *psychological* distress. Do we lead with a compassionate heart and hope that we will utter just the right healing words? Do we offer a verbal "Hail Mary"? The harder we try to improvise and find those perfect words in the moment, the more we possibly fail, or even make things worse.

In this book, we describe the development and guidelines for implementation of a model for providing psychological support to a person in acute psychological distress. Perhaps that person is a friend or family member. Perhaps that person is a coworker.

Perhaps that person is an accident survivor, a survivor of a disaster, or a survivor of a crime. We call this support *psychological first aid* (PFA). Think of it this way, *as physical first aid is to the practice of medicine, psychological first aid is to the practice of psychotherapy.* In this book, we describe one specific model of PFA, the Johns Hopkins RAPID PFA model. It is a unique model in that it is theoretically grounded, evidence-informed, and evidence-based. Research has shown us that this model, or its derivatives, can not only mitigate acute distress but also have positive effects that can endure at least a year.

So, let's start with a little background. The development of the current model does not precisely parallel the general history of PFA, as you will see in chapter 1. So, we will briefly describe how we got here. The evolution of the current model to a large degree reflects the experiences of its developers, one of whom (GSE) is one of the authors of this book. The roots of our PFA model can be found in the community resilience initiatives of the authors in Kuwait after the Gulf War of 1990–91, as well as within the emergence of the relatively new field of disaster mental health (circa 1992).

Our first major attempt at developing crisis-oriented models of psychological support was necessitated by two factors. One was the recognition by the FBI Behavioral Sciences Unit that law enforcement professionals worked in high-stress environments. There was some evidence that if an agent was involved in a shooting, even though physically unharmed, that experience would shorten the career of that agent. The former assistant chief of the FBI Behavioral Sciences Unit was Dr. James Reese, who was a true pioneer. Though most famous for the Unit's seminal research into serial killers, Reese approached me (GSE) to assist with his initiatives to save the careers of FBI agents. I agreed. Reese, together with other agents such as Jim Horn, had developed stress management programs that were very well received. Although formal mental health services (employee assistance, psychological and psychiatric services) were available to the FBI, Reese felt something was missing.

The second factor informing our need to develop a psychological support model was the epidemic of posttraumatic distress after the first Gulf War of 1990–91. The nation of Kuwait lies in a portion of the Arabian Peninsula. It possesses one of two significant natural harbors on the Arabian Gulf, yielding an area long known for its prominence as a mercantile center and for its industrious inhabitants. In 1938, a major oil strike occurred in the Burgan region of Kuwait. In 1946, Kuwait inaugurated its first oil exportation. Needless to say, Kuwait prospered from its petroleum revenues. However, on July 17, 1990, Iraq's Saddam Hussein accused Kuwait of driving down oil prices through overproduction. On August 2, 1990, the Iraqi army invaded Kuwait, occupying the city of Kuwait and the major petroleum-related facilities. In response, United States President George H. W. Bush convened a military coalition to liberate Kuwait. On January 16, 1991, allied forces began the air war, and subsequently a ground campaign, designed to drive Iraqi forces from Kuwait. February 26, 2021, marked the thirtieth anniversary of the liberation of Kuwait from invading Iraqi forces.

In April of 1992, the Amir of Kuwait, Sheikh Jaber Al-Ahmed Al-Sabah established the Social Development Office (SDO) within the Amiri Diwan (Office of His Highness the Amir of Kuwait) to foster the psychological "rehabilitation" of the Kuwaiti people, who had been traumatized from the Iraqi occupation of Kuwait. To this end, the SDO was established under the leadership of Dr. Basheer Al-Rashidi, who was selected as chairman. At the request Dr. Al-Rashidi, as well as former National Institute of Mental Health director Dr. Bertram Brown, I (GSE) was asked to develop clinical training programs for the SDO and was later appointed senior advisor on research to the Amir, serving in the Office of the Amir.

As we looked to develop psychological support programs for law enforcement professionals and for survivors of the Iraqi invasion of Kuwait, we faced two significant barriers: (1) the stigma that was associated with seeking psychological support, and (2) the paucity of clinicians trained to provide emergency psychological support, especially in the field outside of hospital or clinic practice settings. We could not take a traditional "pathology"-oriented approach to the delivery of mental health services, even though posttraumatic stress disorder (PTSD) and posttraumatic depression appeared to be common in law enforcement and virtually epidemic in the Kuwaiti population, appearing at prevalence rates estimated at 10%–15% in law enforcement and 18%–40% in the Kuwaiti population. To attempt to overcome these barriers, we chose to utilize a "resilience" approach to the provision of psychological support. The resilience approach seemed well suited to both situations. Such an approach may be viewed as one that assists people in rebounding from adversity through an emphasis on facilitating adjustment to challenging circumstances, rather than through a pathology-oriented treatment and rehabilitation approach.

We reviewed literature that suggested variations on a theme of psychological crisis intervention delivered by those outside of the mental health professions that might prove useful in our current dilemma. Crisis intervention should not be considered treatment but instead a means of fostering resilience, that is, helping people rebound from adversity, and it must be advertised as such. Perhaps the first solid evidence that a crisis-oriented model might be applicable emerged from the efforts of T. W. Salmon (1919) who made a significant contribution to the literature on nontraditional psychological intervention through his recollections and analyses of interventions with shell shock and the war neuroses during World War I. He observed that acute crisis-oriented interventions were more effective than traditional psychotherapeutics, a finding that would be shown again in the wake of the terrorist attacks of September 11, 2001.

Another significant contribution came from the work of Eric Lindemann (1944) and Gerald Caplan (1964) in community psychiatry after the tragic Cocoanut Grove nightclub fire of November 28, 1942. And the 1960s and 1970s saw the deinstitutionalization of mental health services and the emergence of the community mental health movement. The emergent components of many community mental health centers relied heavily upon community volunteers trained exclusively in psychological crisis intervention. I (GSE) witnessed the effectiveness of this approach firsthand as a community crisis intervention volunteer, having been previously trained in business administration and accounting. Durlak (1979) had shown that basic psychological support (similar to basic physical first aid) could be effectively provided by individuals without prior mental health training. This finding was consistent with the findings of Eisdorpher and Golann (1969) and is consistent with the observations of Levenson (2003), Greenstone (2005), and Castellano (2018), as well as from the Defense Centers of Excellence (2011) and Department of Justice (2019) recommendations to Congress.

Therefore, the decision was made to develop a curriculum and intervention model for acute psychological support for the FBI and for the SDO wherein FBI agents and other law enforcement professionals were instructed in the provision of psychological first aid to the law enforcement profession, and community leaders, educators, medical personnel, fire fighters, and police officers were instructed in the provision of psychological first aid services to the citizens of Kuwait via walk-in clinics and telephone hotlines. These were people who knew the professions, the cultures, and the communities. This model was also adopted by the International Critical Incident Stress Foundation, a United Nations–affiliated nongovernmental organization.

In fairness, it should be said that we did not refer to our curriculum as "psychological first aid," but it did indeed represent the forerunner of what would later become the Johns Hopkins RAPID psychological first aid curriculum, possessing core elements of rapport-building, assessment, triage, mitigation, and follow-up. However, perhaps the most important aspect of our curriculum and psychological intervention model was that it was designed to train persons who had not received previous training in psychology or psychiatry to deliver what might be, due to informal professional, cultural, or logistical barriers, the only informed psychological care incident responders and survivors of disasters might receive. In fact, more than 800 members of the US Department of State (DS), including employees and family members, have been trained in the model and it is considered one of the, if not *the*, largest US Government Peer Support Programs, with representation within every region around the world. The program was developed and structured specifically for the needs of DS.

The Johns Hopkins model described in this book has benefitted from countless revisions and years of relevant research extending far beyond the curriculum. Nevertheless, the roots of the Johns Hopkins RAPID model described in this book can be traced back to vaunted halls of the FBI Behavioral Sciences Unit in Quantico, Virginia, and the sands of the Arabian Peninsula as readily as they can be found in the community mental health movement of the 1960s.

Ironically, my (GSE) tenure in the Amiri Diwan of Kuwait ended in April 2001. On September 11, 2001, the United States experienced terrorist attacks upon the Pentagon near Washington, DC, and upon the two World Trade Center towers in New York City. These attacks would change the world, but they also provided opportunities to continue to develop our emerging model of PFA. Several days after the attacks, both my coauthor and I were asked to train and assist in the implementation of psychological crisis intervention programs. Our efforts were primarily focused on implementing the crisis intervention services with law enforcement personnel who had been adversely affected by the attacks. To reach the large body of law enforcement personnel in the New York and New Jersey area, however, we also trained them to provide "peer psychological support" using the model even though they had little or no previous training in psychology. We realized training needed to be brief and goal directed. A typical crisis intervention might only last 15 to 20 minutes. We ultimately spent three years working with the New York City Police, the New Jersey State Police, the COP 2 COP crisis intervention program now housed at Rutgers University, the Secret Service, and the Port Authority Police of New York and New Jersey.

These last experiences were what ultimately led to the final framework for the Johns Hopkins model that we would implement under the auspices of the Johns Hopkins Bloomberg School of Public Health with partial funding from the US Centers for Disease Control and Prevention (CDC). The model's final form was largely a result of the guidance, support, and contributions of the CDC's principal investigator Jon Links, PhD, along with Cindy Parker, MD, MPH, O. Lee McCabe, PhD, Daniel Barnett, MD, MPH, Natalie Semon, MSEd, and Carol B. Thompson, MS, MBA. Katurah Bland was also of assistance in the administrative aspects of our training programs. Andrea Everly provided the creative materials adapted for the ongoing case study used throughout the book.

The RAPID PFA model contained in this book is the latest version of an intervention process modified significantly beyond the initial model supported by the Centers for Disease Control and Prevention as informed by controlled research, deliberation-based consensus, and continuing field applications. It is a simple, easy-to-learn process wherein you will learn how to establish rapport through reflective listening, assess another person's current level of distress, prioritize response urgency, practice simple techniques to stabilize and mitigate psychological distress, and know when to facilitate access to higher levels of care. We shall also discuss the importance of taking care of yourself (i.e., self-care) as a provider of PFA.

PFA in not psychotherapy nor is it a substitute for psychotherapy. It does not entail diagnosis or treatment. We believe PFA can be an effective public health intervention especially well-suited for areas wherein health care resources are scarce, situations where access to emergent care is limited, or as a means of significantly increasing surge capacity in the wake of organizational or community adversity, such as in the case of disasters and workplace or community violence. It seems especially well suited to enhance community resilience through enhancing community (and organizational) surge capacity using personnel familiar with the indigenous logistics and cultures. Lastly, it might be a way to finally achieve an approximation of universal mental health care at the community level (Everly, 2019).

This book follows a structure that is consistent with the recommendation of Leonardo Da Vinci, who argued that we should first study the science and then practice the art born of that science. The book has three major sections: part I, Psychological First Aid: First, Study the Science; part II, Psychological First Aid: Practicing the Art; and part III, Psychological First Aid: Further Considerations. In part I, we review the definitions, core concepts, research, and historical development of PFA. We also review the psychological consequences of trauma and disaster. This review is designed to set expectations of the most prevalent adverse reactions a provider is likely to encounter in the field. Similarly, the review may provide an empirical rationale for the development and implementation of PFA programs.

In part II, we explain the practice of PFA. We take a step-by-step approach to the instruction of the Johns Hopkins RAPID PFA model. Within each of the *practice* chapters, we employ a structure wherein each practice component is defined, its development reviewed, putative mechanisms of action discussed, and only then do we provide implementation guidelines.

Part III extends our discussion into the critical areas of PFA with new chapters on the application of PFA with children, PFA and cultural diversity, and community-based PFA to expand psychological support services not only in disaster but perhaps as the only feasible means of approximating universal mental health care. Lastly, we address the important issue of self-care.

There is a Key Point Summary at the end of each chapter, and an additional unique feature of the book is that we provide a trauma-related case study that thematically unifies each chapter by demonstrating each chapter's operative component in an ongoing PFA intervention scenario. It is relevant to note that this is a pre-COVID-19 scenario.

The online learning platform Coursera offers introductory training in the Johns Hopkins RAPID PFA model (https://www.coursera.org /learn/psychological-first-aid). As this book is being written, more than 425,000 people have enrolled in that course from around the globe. Indeed, a recent article in the prestigious *Scientific American* recommended that "everyone" should take the Coursera online class (Editors, 2021).

In the spirit of full disclosure, we acknowledge that the fields of psychological crisis intervention and disaster mental health, within which PFA is considered an essential component, continue to evolve as new experiences shape our understanding and practice. It was the observation of former director of the National Institute of Mental Health Dr. Bertram Brown that these fields are fraught with the lack of a standard nomenclature and a contentiousness that serves to make an already intrinsically challenging pursuit even more difficult. It is hoped that this second edition will continue to bring clarity, and perhaps compassion, to these muddled and often misunderstood fields.

References

Caplan, G. (1964). *Principles of preventive psychiatry.* New York, NY: Basic Books.

Castellano, C. (2018). Silver award: Reciprocal peer support for addressing mental health crises among police, veterans, mothers of special needs children, and others. 2018 APA Psychiatric Services Achievement Awards. *Psychiatric Services, 69,* e7–8. http://dx.doi.org/10.1176/appi.ps.691006.

Defense Centers of Excellence (2011). *Best practices identified for peer support programs.* Washington, DC: Defense Centers of Excellence.

Department of Justice, Community Oriented Policing Services. (2019). *Law enforcement mental health and wellness act: Report to Congress.* Washington, DC: US Department of Justice.

Durlak, J. (1979). Comparative effectiveness of paraprofessional and professional helpers. *Psychological Bulletin, 86,* 80–92. http://dx.doi.org/10.1037/0033-2909.86.1.80.

Editors. (2021, February). A step to ease the pandemic mental health crisis. *Scientific American, 324,* 10. http://doi.org/10.1038/scientificamerican0221-10.

Eisdorpher, C., & Golann, S. (1969). Principles for the training of "new professionals" in mental health. *Community Mental Health Journal, 5,* 349–357. http://dx.doi.org/10.1007/BF01438980.

Everly, G. S., Jr. (2020). Psychological first aid (PFA) to expand mental health support and foster resiliency in underserved and access-compromised areas. *Crisis, Stress, and Human Resilience, 1,* 227–232.

Greenstone, J. L. (2005). Peer support for police hostage and crisis negotiators. *Journal of Police Crisis Negotiations, 5,* 45–55. http://dx.doi.org/10.1300/J173v05n01_05.

Levenson, R. (2003). Peer support in law enforcement. *International Journal of Emergency Mental Health, 5,* 147–152.

Lindemann, E. (1944). Symptomatology and management of acute grief. *American Journal of Psychiatry, 101,* 141–148. http://dx.doi.org/10.1176/ajp.101.2.141.

Salmon, T. (1919). War neuroses and their lesson. *New York Medical Journal, 108,* 993–994.

ACKNOWLEDGMENTS

THIS BOOK IS A CULMINATION of numerous and diverse experiences spanning four decades. Thus, those who influenced the final product are many. Most noteworthy are my intellectual mentors Theodore Millon, PhD, DSc, and David C. McClelland, PhD, at Harvard University; Jeffery T. Mitchell, PhD, at the University of Maryland, from whom I learned how to apply structure to chaos; Cindy Parker, MD, MPH, Daniel Barnett, MD, MPH, and Natalie Semon, MSEd, at the Johns Hopkins Bloomberg School of Public Health who helped me transition from clinician to public health scholar; O. Lee McCabe, PhD, Karen Swartz, MD, and James "Jimmy" Potash, MD, MPH, at the Johns Hopkins School of Medicine who have provided ongoing support and encouragement to disaster psychiatry at Johns Hopkins; Michael J. Kaminsky, MD, MBA, at the Johns Hopkins School of Medicine, who was referred to by his colleagues as "a psychiatrist's psychiatrist." He was the best disaster psychiatrist with whom I've ever worked. His journey ended far too soon. And lastly, Jon Links, PhD, also at the Johns Hopkins Bloomberg School of Public Health, to whom I will forever be indebted for igniting and nurturing my professional renaissance. Thank you! (GSE)

I thank Stephen Bono, PhD, for his close to thirty years of mentoring and friendship. I also thank Mark Danzig, United States Department of State Bureau of Diplomatic Security Senior Advisor and Peer Support Director; Claudine Meyer-Sager, Head CISM at Skyguide, the Swiss Air Navigation Services; Allan McDougall, former International Director of the Emergency Response Team (ERT) of the United Steelworkers (USW), author, and current Client Relations Coordinator for the law firm of Provost and Umphrey; and Duronda Pope, current Director of the ERT of the USW for your inspiration, passion, and persistence in advancing the application of psychological first aid, and for allowing me to be a part of your truly remarkable communities. Thanks also to my remarkable colleagues and friends at Loyola University Maryland. Most importantly, I thank my family, including our newest addition Leo, for always providing grounding, comfort, support, and a place to call home. (JML)

We wish to thank O. Lee McCabe, PhD, at the Johns Hopkins School of Medicine and the Johns Hopkins Bloomberg School of Public Health who has been one of the most professionally and personally influential people we have ever known. We also thank Michael J. Klag, MD, MPH, former Dean, Johns Hopkins Bloomberg School of Public Health, for his support of the initiatives that led to the RAPID PFA model and to the first edition of this book. Thanks also to Andrea N. Everly (Harvard University) for providing the creative foundation for the applied case used throughout the book. A special thanks to Grace Homany for her editorial assistance on this edition.

We also thank Robin W. Coleman, Adelene Jane Medrano, Juliana McCarthy, and Hilary Jacqmin from Johns Hopkins University Press, as well as freelance copyeditor Joanne Haines, for their willingness to adopt the text, their patience throughout the project, and their editorial and marketing assistance.

PSYCHOLOGICAL FIRST AID

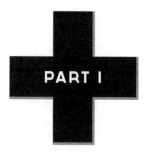

FIRST, STUDY THE SCIENCE

In this first part of the book, we trace the history and meaning of psychological first aid (PFA). In addition, we introduce the Johns Hopkins RAPID model of PFA. We then review relevant research associated with the practice of PFA. Finally, we review the psychological and behavioral consequences of trauma and disaster.

ONE | Psychological First Aid

Definition, History, and Foundational Research

ACCORDING TO THE UNITED NATIONS, "Mental health has large intrinsic value as it relates to the core of what makes us human," thus anything that threatens the mental health of large numbers of people threatens the core fabric of society itself (United Nations, 2020, p. 5). Most readers of this book have directly observed another human being in psychological distress, whether it was friend, a family member, a coworker, or perhaps a stranger. Similarly, those of us who have observed someone in distress have usually been motivated to offer some form of support to attempt to ease the suffering we witnessed. Sometimes our efforts were effective and sometimes they were not. Sometimes, despite our best efforts, our actions appeared to make matters worse, seeming to intensify acute distress. At times such as these we lamented the absence of a psychological "magic bullet," a verbal "Hail Mary," that would immediately end the suffering and lead to the realization of the promise we made that "everything will be OK." Consistent with our intuitions, a recommendation in the *American Journal of Psychiatry* states that "shortly after a traumatic event, it is important that those affected be provided, in an empath-

3

ic manner, practical, pragmatic psychological support" (Bisson et al., 2007, p. 1017). Lucky for us and in lieu of an impossible magic bullet, over the last 100 years there has evolved what we now refer to as *psychological first aid* (PFA).

Defining Psychological First Aid

Perhaps the best way to conceptualize PFA is as the mental health analogue to physical first aid. PFA may be simply defined as a supportive and compassionate presence designed to stabilize and mitigate acute distress, as well as facilitate access to continued care. PFA does not entail diagnosis, nor does it entail treatment. PFA is a tactical variation within the 100-year-old field of psychological crisis intervention. In this book we describe the Johns Hopkins RAPID model of PFA. The goals of this model of PFA are:

1. to meet basic needs;
2. to stabilize acute psychological and/or behavioral reactions;
3. to mitigate acute distress, impairment, or dysfunction to assist in the recovery of some degree of adaptive functionality (resilience);
4. to foster natural coping and resilience mechanisms; and
5. to facilitate access to continued support or higher-level care, but only if indicated.

To achieve these goals, the Johns Hopkins RAPID PFA model relies on five distinct steps, or phases. **RAPID** is an acronym that denotes the model's constituent phases:

R — Rapport and reflective listening. Effective psychological crisis intervention is predicated on gaining rapport with the person in distress. Consider rapport as a form of interpersonal connectedness that serves as a platform for the remaining aspects of the model. Reflective listening techniques facilitate the attainment of rapport quickly and effectively.

A — Assessment. The term *assessment* is used liberally here and consists of screening (Is there any evidence of need for PFA or other types of intervention?) and appraisal (What is the severity or gravity of need?). This information is generated, not through the use psychological tests or mental status examinations, but rather through the process of listening to the person's story of distress. The story consists of what happened (the stressor event) and the person's reactions (signs and symptoms) in response to the event. There is no need to ask the person to relive the incident, rather only a context is sought. Of far greater importance is the person's reaction to the incident. This becomes the focus of the intervention.

P — Prioritization. Having heard the story, you must determine how urgent the need is for intervention. This becomes an exercise in psychological triage. As mentioned above, this phase results from the processes of screening and appraisal. As a public health intervention model especially well-suited for disaster mental health response, RAPID gives emphasis to the process of psychological triage by making it a discrete step in the model.

I — Intervention. Having heard the story and the associated reactions, some efforts toward stabilization and mitigation of adverse reactions is often recommended, if not expected. We shall review numerous practical crisis intervention techniques you can use. This step in the model is a key differentiator that separates the RAPID PFA model from many other PFA models. Many other models of PFA rely on three simple mechanisms: listen, protect, refer. Our approach is to view PFA as a "force multiplier" where its utilization serves to expand mental health support capacity. In disaster settings, the listen-protect-refer approach will usually prove inadequate. Similarly, if we are to approximate universal mental health access at the community level, models of PFA with intervention intention beyond listen-protect-refer will be needed. This will be covered in more detail in a later chapter. Thus, the RAPID model of PFA employs more "mechanisms of action" (active ingredients) than most other models of PFA, including but not limited to anticipatory guidance (setting expectation), explanatory guidance (positing explanations for the felt reactions), prescriptive guidance (stress management), and even cognitive reframing.

D—Disposition. Having heard the story and responded with an appropriate intervention, you now must determine what to do next. "Where do we go from here?" is a question you should ask yourself and might even ask the person you've assisted. Most behavioral outcomes are recovery or referral to some alternative source of support. We shall delineate guidelines for both.

As statistician George Box once famously said, "All models are approximations. Essentially, all models are wrong, but some are useful" (Box & Draper, 1987, p. 424). We believe the RAPID model of PFA is this type of model. Models are representations. RAPID is a heuristic mnemonic representation of the fundamental needs and corollary compensatory processes of the human mind in crisis. The Johns Hopkins RAPID PFA model is, however, unique in that it is theory-driven, evidence-informed, and empirically validated at the individual, group, and community levels. Therefore, it is an innovative model of PFA.

Development of the PFA Concept

To paraphrase philosopher and historian George Santayana, those who fail to read history are doomed to repeat it, or as it pertains to the current context, to reinvent it. So, let's take a quick history lesson as it pertains to PFA in general. PFA is the integration of two conceptual and practical foundations: (1) physical first aid and (2) psychological crisis intervention.

Regarding physical first aid, we must go back a thousand years. The Order of St. John may be the first organized effort to practice and disseminate physical first aid. The Order was founded in 1048 in Jerusalem with the intention of training laypeople to provide medical first aid care to travelers and victims of the battlefield. The mission of the Knights of St. John enjoyed varying success during and after the Crusades. The next major advance in physical first aid would not come for centuries later. In 1859, Henry Dunant, a Swiss businessman, was shocked at the aftermath of the battle of Solferino, Italy, which reportedly left 40,000 dead or injured (Boissier, 1985). Seeing the horror, he enlisted the aid of local villagers to provide medical first aid to battlefield casualties. Several years later, his efforts, along with others, led to the creation of the International Red Cross for which he shared the first Nobel Peace Prize in 1901. Within this formative process, the term *first aid* is said to have been used for the first time, perhaps as early as 1863 (Boissier, 1985). Extending physical first aid beyond the battlefield, the Industrial Revolution saw the rise of ambulance services in Great Britain, such as St. John Ambulance. They provided physical first aid and transportation for such injured workers as miners, police, and transport workers. Ernest Hemingway famously served as a civilian ambulance driver on the Italian front during World War I. The story of psychological crisis intervention begins much later. According to one of the early writers in the field of psychological crisis intervention, "A little help, rationally directed and purposely focused at a strategic time, is more effective than extensive help given at a period of less emotional accessibility" (Rapoport, 1965, p. 30). Later, Swanson and Carbon (1989), writing for the American Psychiatric Association Task Force Report on the Treatment of Psychiatric Disorders, stated, "Crisis intervention is a proven approach to helping in the pain of an emotional crisis" (p. 2520).

The field of psychological crisis intervention can be traced back more than 100 years to the management of "shell shock" in World War I. Traditional psychotherapeutic interventions consistently failed to assist soldiers in regaining functional capacities subsequent to combat-related psychological crises and injury. Dr. T. S. Salmon observed that the English and French medical corps had therefore altered their approach to treating the various battlefield and traumatic neuroses by moving their psychiatric facilities to more forward positions near the sound of the artillery. They utilized stabilization, brief support, and mitigation procedures. He argued that the American hospitals should do the same. As a result of these changes, he observed a dramatic increase in the return-to-duty rates achieved by the end of the war (Artiss, 1963).

This new approach to psychological intervention consisted of three core principles (Artiss, 1963): (1) proximity, (2) immediacy, and (3) expectancy (P-I-E). The P-I-E principles were subsequently shown to be effective on the battlefield for reducing posttraumatic casualties (Salmon, 1919; Solomon & Benbenishty, 1986; Solomon, Shklar, & Mikulincer, 2005). P-I-E not only represents the defining characteristics of psychological crisis intervention but is what differentiates it from psychotherapy. So, what is P-I-E?

P — Proximity. From its origins in military psychiatry, proximity referred to the provision of acute psychological support in, or very close to, the field of combat. The civilian variant would entail providing crisis intervention services in the community away from a hospital or clinic setting. It would especially include mobile crisis services. Thus, proximity is a form of static (e.g., walk-in crisis centers or shelters located throughout a community) or dynamic (e.g., mobile crisis units) outreach.

I — Immediacy. Immediacy refers to the urgency provision of psychological support as predicated by the emergence of need (i.e., the emergence of signs and symptoms of distress). Immediacy is not defined in terms of temporal proximity to an event, per se, but the deployment of crisis teams can certainly be enacted based upon the occurrence of a significant incident alone. No matter what, teams are encouraged to perform surveillance prior to active intervention.

E — Expectancy. Expectancy refers to the view that the current state of psychological disequilibrium is an adjustment reaction representing a current perturbation from one's usual ability to function. Therefore, the goal of intervention is to address that current adjustment reaction, not cure any pre-existing psychiatric syndrome, even if it is present. The expectancy principle serves to depathologize acute psychological distress. In doing so it may serve to begin to foster a sense of resilience by creating a self-fulfilling prophecy of self-efficacy and resilience.

Another contribution to the development of psychological crisis intervention emerged during World War II but not on the battlefield. In fact, it served to temporarily take the nation's focus off World War II. The Cocoanut Grove was the most popular nightclub in Boston in 1942.

It was a favorite retreat for military personnel and sports enthusiasts. On the evening of November 28, 1942, it would become the scene of the deadliest nightclub fire in American history. That evening, the nightclub was dangerously overcrowded with more than 1,000 patrons. The club was reportedly licensed to hold 460. A fire started inside around 10:15 p.m. and spread rapidly. Sadly, many exits were either obscured or locked. Other doors opened inward, thus trapping patrons trying to open the doors to escape. In the end, 492 people died and 166 were injured. The fire was not only traumatic for those in attendance but also for the entire community. Eric Lindemann's study (1944) of the trajectory of the grief process subsequent to that catastrophic fire made a significant contribution to community resilience and acute psychological intervention research. Lindemann chronicled the recovery process as being contingent upon what he called "grief work." Anchored in the work of Sigmund Freud, grief work was defined as the "emancipation from the bondage to the deceased" (Lindemann, 1944, p. 190). This notion of a natural grief trajectory was widely accepted despite little evidence of its necessity. Lindemann was later joined by Gerald Caplan (1964) in the creation of a community mental health program that emphasized community outreach and crisis intervention in the Boston metropolitan area. This served as a model for many other communities across the United States.

The 1960s and 1970s heralded the advent of the formalized community mental health movement. In general, mental health care was decentralized. Large psychiatric institutions were closed, replaced by a proliferation of community mental health centers. The outreach and emergent care component of the community mental health movement often relied on telephone crisis hotlines and walk-in crisis clinics most commonly staffed by paraprofessionals, peer counselors, and other community volunteers. Research argued for the viability of a community-based psychological crisis intervention capacity that relied primarily on paraprofessionals, a focus ultimately championed by Dr. Bertram Brown, assistant surgeon general of the United States. Later, "peer" crisis intervention teams (as differentiated from mental health clinicians) were established in organizations whose employees were deemed at high risk for psychological distress and injury. It has been shown that these "peer" crisis interventions can be as effective as mental health clinicians in providing acute psychological support (Castellano, 2018; Defense Centers of Excellence, 2011; Durlak, 1979; Eisdorpher & Golann, 1969). These community-based intervention initiatives proved effective in reducing psychiatric cases, facilitating access to more traditional psychological care when needed and sustaining adherence during treatment (Bordow & Porritt, 1979; Bunn & Clarke, 1979; Caplan, 1964; Decker & Stubblebine, 1972; Langsley, Machotka, & Flomenhaft, 1971; Parad & Parad, 1968).

We mentioned earlier that the work of Salmon (1919) and Artiss (1963) helped delineate the tactical differences between crisis intervention and psychotherapy as being embedded in the P-I-E concept. Similarly, Israeli psychologist Zahava Solomon (Solomon & Benbenishty, 1986) investigated the core crisis intervention principles of "proximity, immediacy, and expectancy." Consistent with the seminal observations of her predecessors, Solomon found that when P-I-E was applied in the field to aid Israeli soldiers, it was effective in reducing acute psychological distress. Of the three operative constructs, expectancy appeared to be the most effective. Most importantly, however, are the implications of a 20-year longitudinal study by Solomon, Shklar, and Mikulincer (2005) that evaluated the long-term effectiveness of frontline P-I-E provided to the combat stress reaction casualties 20 years earlier. Using a longitudinal quasi-experimental design, combat stress reaction casualties of the 1982 Lebanon War who received frontline treatment were compared to comparable combat stress reaction casualties who did not receive frontline treatment and other soldiers who did not experience combat stress reaction. Twenty years after the war, traumatized soldiers who received frontline psychological crisis intervention, following the core principles of proximity, immediacy, expectancy, had lower rates of posttraumatic and psychiatric symptoms and reported better social functioning than similarly exposed soldiers who did not receive frontline intervention. The cumulative effect of the core crisis principles was documented in that the more principles applied, the stronger the effect. The authors concluded, "Frontline treatment is associated with improved outcomes even two decades after its application. This treatment may also be effective for nonmilitary precursors of posttraumatic stress disorder" (Solomon, Shklar, & Mikulincer, 2005, p. 2309).

By 1990, psychological crisis intervention was being applied to large-scale disasters, assisting not only emergency responders but also civilians. The British Psychological Society (1990) argued that psychological crisis intervention had reached a level of development that its tactical constituents needed to be organized better strategically. The Society wrote that psychological crisis intervention, and one would think especially disaster response, should consist of an integrated continuum of care. The American Red Cross embraced this notion in the development of its disaster response training in 1992. In fact, the first author of this book (GSE) was tasked with developing the American Red Cross disaster mental health response team for the state of Maryland.

By 1992, arguably the most popular psychological crisis interventions were a constellation of interventions within the rubric referred to as Critical Incident Stress Management (CISM; see Everly & Mitchell, 1997). CISM is best viewed as an integrated, multicomponent continuum of emergent psychological support that has been shown to be effective in mitigating adverse psychological reactions after a disaster (Boscarino, Adams, & Figley, 2005). However, one of its component tactical interventions, a form of group crisis intervention, a *critical incident stress debriefing* (CISD) — often referred to simply as *debriefing* or PD (*psychological debriefing*) for short — had found favor as perhaps the most widely used single crisis intervention of that era. It should be clarified that CISD is a semistructured *group* crisis intervention originally designed solely for use by functional workgroups of emergency services personnel. CISD was unfortunately commonly confused with CISM. It is suggested that CISD, because of its purported success and somewhat liberal definitions early in its development, began to be implemented beyond the scope of its intended applications. The widespread use and purported success of CISD demanded scrutiny to assess context suitability and overall effectiveness, despite the logistical difficulty and even the ethical dilemma of using a control group while conducting field research with traumatized persons during disasters and related events.

The subsequent research initiatives may have done more harm than good according to some authors, however, as early efforts could only offer approximations of the actual interventions of interest (British Psychological Society, 2015; Hawker, Durkin, & Hawker, 2010; Regel & Dyregrov, 2012; Tuckey, 2007). These approximations were understandably criticized for lacking both internal and external validity (British Psychological Society, 2015; Regel & Dyregrov, 2012; Tamrakar, Murphy, & Elklit, 2019; Tuckey, 2007). Nevertheless, reviews of the overall effectiveness of CISD/PD were attempted with these low fidelity approximations and subsequently published as a Cochrane Review (Rose et al., 2002). The publication of the Cochrane Review led to concerns of the effectiveness of standalone "individual debriefings" (debriefings done with individuals rather than groups) in medical settings. This rebuke might be warranted for the acute medical populations that were represented in the Cochrane sample but remain irrelevant to the use of "group debriefings" applied to emergency responders, which, as noted, was the intention of the creators of the CISD/PFA methodology.

Well-intended, but arguably methodologically flawed (British Psychological Society, 2015; Dyregrov & Regel, 2012; Everly & Mitchell, 2000; Regel & Dyregrov, 2012), efforts to assess the effectiveness of CISD/PD led to many misconceptions and inappropriate conclusions regarding early psychological intervention (psychological crisis intervention) in general, and PD in particular. These misconceptions seemed to be self-sustaining and reached the stature of urban mythology according to Atle Dyregrov and Stephen Regel, international authorities in the field (Dyregrov & Regel, 2012; Regel & Dyregrov, 2012), as well as others (British Psychological Society, 2015; Hawker, Durkin, & Hawker, 2010; Tuckey, 2007). According to Dyregrov and Regel (2012), much of the misunderstanding and subsequent debates around CISD/PD are based on two studies (i.e., Bisson et al., 1997 and Hobbs et al., 1996):

> Both studies have since been demonstrated not only to have methodological flaws, but also not to have given adequate training to those carrying out the PD interventions. . . . This inevitably has caused significant confusion not only in terminology, but also in the areas of research, practice, and policy. This lack of clarity and understanding in the terminology surrounding early interventions has subsequently influenced the literature on what works best and for whom, and confusion in this area has reigned for over a decade. (p. 272)

The findings of the British Psychological Society (2015) echo the aforementioned:

> The debriefing debate has been raging ever since the publication of the Cochrane Review. As has been argued cogently by colleagues in the chapters above, it seems that the findings of this review are fundamentally flawed. . . . No wonder, then, that these studies produced the results that they did, no wonder that the Cochrane Review's findings reported what they did, and no wonder still that the misleading press coverage and knee jerk responses that led to the blanket bans on its use that emerged subsequently. (p. 70)

In a recent commentary and review, Tamrakar, Murphy, and Elklit (2019) concluded that the influential Cochrane Reviews, which summarized and evaluated "debriefings," violated its own reporting guidelines. The authors note, "The studies included in the Cochrane Review . . . are in violation with four out of the five aspects of the integrity of CISD/PD as an intervention as per the Cochrane Handbook" (Tamrakar, Murphy, & Elklit, 2019, p. 50). Subsequent publication of data from randomized investigations with higher internal validity and fidelity to original models are supportive of CISM (Boscarino, Adams, & Figley, 2005, 2011) and group crisis intervention, specifically CISD/PD (Adler et al., 2008; Adler et al., 2009; Deahl et al., 2000; Tuckey & Scott, 2014).

As is often the case in any nascent field, there is eagerness to bring innovation to application, which may lead to resistance, spirited debate, and even issues of professional territoriality. As Martin Deahl noted over 20 years ago, "The effectiveness of acute interventions . . . has become increasingly politicized and more than a matter of science" (2000, p. 931). In apparent agreement, Atle Dyregrov (1998) concluded:

> In my opinion the debate on debriefing is not only a scientific but also a political debate. It entails power and positions in the therapeutic world . . . many people being trained in the technique were peer support personnel and mental health workers outside psychiatric institutions. [Debriefing] thus has been partly self-help and consumer driven where the recipients of services have had more control than in traditional academic or medical approaches. (p. 7)

Now, 30 years after the birth of the field of disaster mental health, some of these issues may persist, but overall we seem to be reaching a better understanding of the who, what, when, where, and how of acute psychological intervention.

Rapprochement

Based upon the research cited above, as well as an appreciation of the importance of early psychological intervention, the current perspective dominating the field of early psychological interventions after trauma and disaster is to proceed cautiously. But at the same time there has appeared a demand, if not desperation, for some form of psychological crisis intervention. After the terrorist attacks of September 11, 2001, interest in PFA was rekindled and the modern era of PFA began. The emergence of the 2020–21 COVID-19 pandemic, vitriolic political discord, and social unrest in the United States has added to this desperation. The United Nations (2020) correctly predicted a surge of psychological distress, a "hidden pandemic" of sorts, wherein millions of people would be adversely affected by stress, trauma, and burnout as a result. Vicarious trauma and burnout were expected and subsequently realized within emergency services and health care professionals:

> First responders and frontline workers, particularly workers in health and long-term care . . . are under exceptional stress, being faced with extreme workloads, difficult decisions, risks of becoming infected and spreading infection to families and communities and witnessing deaths of patients. Stigmatization of these workers is common in too many communities. There have been reports of suicide attempts and suicide death by health-care workers. (United Nation, 2020, p. 11)

Given the importance of crisis intervention to human health, and the methodological challenges noted in its initial inquiry, it seems important to continue to scrutinize and assess psychological crisis intervention and disaster mental health initiatives. While randomized controlled trials (RCTs) can add to our knowledge, they should not be the only source of information to inform practice and policy. The conclusion of Regel (2007) that RCTs are not the *sine qua non* of evidence-based medicine seems to be a reasonable conclusion. Former president of the American Psychological Association Martin Seligman (1995) has advocated for the power of nonrandomized quasi-experimental and even pre-experimental designs. He notes, "I have come to believe that the 'effectiveness' study of how patients fare under the actual conditions . . . in the field, can yield . . . 'empirical validation' " (Seligman, 1995, p. 966).

This type of analytic flexibility appears to have been specifically applied to PFA practices. Despite the fact that the review conducted by Fox et al. (2013) for the Advisory Council of the American Red Cross Disaster Services revealed no controlled trials (RCTs or quasi-experimental) supporting the practice of PFA, the authors nevertheless concluded, "Sufficient evidence for psychological first aid is widely supported by available objective observations and expert opinion and best fits the category of 'evidence informed' but without proof of effectiveness" (p. 247). Using the same criteria, there appears to be more than sufficient evidence supporting psychological crisis intervention, debriefing, and related practices, as they serve as background for the development of PFA.

Finally, in their 2009 report published by the World Health Organization, Bisson and Lewis (2009) were unable to find empirical data supporting the use of PFA post disaster or trauma. Nevertheless, the authors note:

> In summary, there is an absence of direct evidence for the effectiveness of PFA, but indirect evidence supports the delivery of services based on the principles of PFA in the first few weeks after a traumatic event. We agree that when delivered PFA should be consistent with research evidence on risk and resilience following trauma; applicable and practical in field settings; appropriate for developmental levels across the lifespan; and culturally informed and delivered in a flexible manner. (p. 15)

The recommendations of Bisson and Lewis (2009) seem prudent. Perhaps we should embrace these recommendations for not only PFA but all psychological crisis interventions, disaster mental health, and related practices as we continue to add to the empirical database.

KEY POINT SUMMARY

1. Psychological first aid (PFA) is a form of psychological crisis intervention.

2. Psychological crisis intervention has over 100 years of application and research supporting its effectiveness. The American Psychiatric Association Task Force Report on the Treatment of Psychiatric Disorders noted, "Crisis intervention is a proven approach to helping in the pain of an emotional crisis" (Swanson & Carbon, 1989, p. 2520).

3. PFA may be thought of as the mental health analogue to physical first aid. It may be simply defined as a supportive and compassionate presence designed to stabilize and mitigate acute distress. PFA is neither diagnosis nor treatment.

4. PFA may be effectively implemented by mental health clinicians, physicians, nurses, educators, emergency services personnel, clergy, and other members of a community.

5. The Johns Hopkins RAPID is one model of PFA especially suited for large-scale public health applications, such as disasters.

6. The goals of RAPID PFA (discussed throughout this book), are the following:

   a. To meet basic needs (medical stability, safety, food, water, shelter).

   b. To stabilize acute psychological and/or behavioral reactions.

   c. To mitigate acute distress, impairment, or dysfunction to assist in recovering some degree of adaptive functionality (resilience).

   d. To foster natural coping and resilience mechanisms.

   e. To facilitate access to continued support, or higher-level care, if indicated.

7. The Johns Hopkins RAPID PFA model relies upon five distinct steps, or phases:

   a. R—Rapport through reflective listening.

   b. A—Assessment. The term *assessment* is used liberally here and consists of two decision points: (1) screening (is there any evidence of need for PFA or other types of intervention) and (2) appraisal (what is the severity or gravity of need), which leads to the next phase in the model.

   c. P—Prioritization. This is an exercise in psychological triage.

   d. I—Intervention. Here, timely and practical crisis intervention techniques, such as anticipatory guidance, explanatory guidance, and prescriptive guidance, are applied to reduce acute distress.

   e. D—Disposition. This phase consists of making a plan to facilitate recovery or referral.

References

Adler, A., Bliese, P. D., McGurk, D., Hoge, C. W., & Castro, C. A. (2009). Battlemind debriefing and battlemind training as early interventions with soldiers returning from Iraq: Randomization by platoon. *Journal of Consulting and Clinical Psychology, 77*, 928–940. http://dx.doi.org/10.1037/a0016877.

Adler, A, Litz, B. T., Castro, C. A., Suvak, M., Thomas, J. L., Burrell, L., & Bliese, P. D. (2008). A group randomized trial of critical incident stress debriefing provided to US peacekeepers. *Journal of Traumatic Stress, 21*, 253–263. http://dx.doi.org/10.1002/jts.20342.

Artiss, K. (1963). Human behavior under stress: From combat to social psychiatry. *Military Medicine, 128*, 1011–1015.

Bisson, J. I., Brayne, M., Ochberg, F., & Everly, G. S., Jr. (2007). Early psychosocial intervention following traumatic events. *American Journal of Psychiatry, 164*, 1016–1019. http://dx.doi.org/10.1176/ajp.2007.164.7.1016.

Bisson, J. I., Jenkins, P., Alexander, J., & Bannister, C. (1997). Randomized controlled trial of psychological debriefings for victims of acute burn trauma. *British Journal of Psychiatry, 171*, 78–81. http://dx.doi.org/10.1192/bjp.171.1.78.

Bisson, J. I., & Lewis, C. (2009). *Systematic review of psychological first aid.* Commissioned by the World Health Organization. Geneva, Switzerland: World Health Organization.

Boissier, P. (1985). *History of the International Committee of the Red Cross. Vol. 1. From Solferino to Tsushima.* Geneva, Switzerland: ICRC.

Bordow, S., & Porritt, D. (1979). An experimental evaluation of crisis intervention. *Social Science and Medicine, 13*, 251–256. http://dx.doi.org/10.1016/0271-7123(79)90042-7.

Boscarino J. A., Adams R. E., & Figley, C. R. (2005). A prospective cohort study of the effectiveness of employer-sponsored crisis interventions after a major disaster. *International Journal of Emergency Mental Health, 7*, 9–22.

Boscarino, J., Adams, R., & Figley, C. (2011). Mental health service use after the World Trade Center disaster: Utilization trends and comparative effectiveness. *Journal of Nervous and Mental Disease, 199*, 91–99. http://dx.doi.org/10.1097/NMD.0b013e3182043b39.

Box, G. E. P., & Draper, N. R. (1987). *Empirical model-building and response surfaces.* New York, NY: John Wiley & Sons.

British Psychological Society Working Party. (1990). *Psychological aspects of disaster.* Leicester, UK: British Psychological Society.

British Psychological Society. (2015). *Early interventions for trauma*. Leicester, UK: British Psychological Society

Bunn, T., & Clarke, A. (1979). Crisis intervention: An experimental study of the effects of a brief period of counselling on the anxiety of relatives of seriously injured or ill hospital patients. *British Journal of Medical Psychology*, 52, 191–195. http://dx.doi.org/10.1111/j.2044-8341.1979.tb02514.x.

Caplan, G. (1964). *Principles of preventive psychiatry*. New York, NY: Basic Books.

Castellano, C. (2018). Silver award: Reciprocal peer support for addressing mental health crises among police, veterans, mothers of special needs children, and others. 2018 APA Psychiatric Services Achievement Awards. *Psychiatric Services*, 69, e7-8. http://dx.doi.org/10.1176/appi.ps.691006.

Deahl, M. (2000). Psychological debriefing: Controversy and challenge. *Australian & New Zealand Journal of Psychiatry*, 34, 929–939. https://doi.org/10.1080/000486700267.

Deahl, M., Srinivasan, M., Jones, N., Thomas, J., Neblett, C., & Jolly, A. (2000). Preventing psychological trauma in soldiers. The role of operational stress training and psychological debriefing. *British Journal of Medical Psychology*, 73, 77–85. http://dx.doi.org/10.1348/000711200160318.

Decker, J., & Stubblebine, J. (1972). Crisis intervention and prevention of psychiatric disability: A follow-up study. *American Journal of Psychiatry*, 129, 725–729. http://dx.doi.org/10.1176/ajp.129.6.725.

Defense Centers of Excellence (2011). *Best practices identified for peer support programs*. Washington, DC: Defense Centers of Excellence.

Durlak, J. (1979). Comparative effectiveness of paraprofessional and professional helpers. *Psychological Bulletin*, 86, 80–92. http://dx.doi.org/10.1037/0033-2909.86.1.80.

Dyregrov, A. (1998). Psychological debriefing — An effective method? *Traumatology*, 4(2). http://dx.doi.org/10.1177/153476569800400203.

Dyregrov, A., & Regel, S. (2012). Early interventions following exposure to traumatic events: Implications for practice from recent research. *Journal of Loss and Trauma*, 17, 271–291. http://dx.doi.org/10.1080/15325024.2011.616832.

Editors. (2021, February). A step to ease the pandemic mental health crisis. *Scientific American*, 324, 10. http://doi.org/10.1038/scientificamerican0221-10.

Eisdorpher, C., & Golann, S. (1969). Principles for the training of "new professionals" in mental health. *Community Mental Health Journal*, 5, 349–357. http://dx.doi.org/10.1007/BF01438980.

Everly, G. S., Jr., & Mitchell, J. T. (1997). *Critical incident stress management (CISM): A new era and standard of care in crisis intervention.* Ellicott City, MD: Chevron.

Everly, G. S., Jr., & Mitchell, J. T. (2000). The debriefing controversy and crisis intervention: A review of lexical and substantive issues. *International Journal of Emergency Mental Health, 2,* 211–225.

Fox, J. H., Burkle, F. M., Jr., Bass, J., Pia, F. A., Epstein, J. L., & Markenson, D. (2013). The effectiveness of psychological first aid as a disaster intervention tool: Research analysis of peer-reviewed literature from 1990–2010. *Disaster Medicine and Public Health Preparedness, 6,* 247–252. http://dx .doi.org/10.1001/dmp.2012.39.

Hawker, D. M., Durkin, J., & Hawker, D. S. J. (2010). To debrief or not to debrief our heroes: That is the question. *Clinical Psychology and Psychotherapy,* Advance online publication. http://dx.doi.org/10.1002/cpp.730.

Hobbs, M., Mayou, R., Harrison, B., & Worlock, P. (1996). A randomised controlled trial of psychological debriefing for victims of road traffic accidents. *British Medical Journal, 313,* 1438–1439. http://dx.doi.org/10.1136/bmj .313.7070.1438.

Langsley, D., Machotka, P., & Flomenhaft, K. (1971). Avoiding mental health admission: A follow-up. *American Journal of Psychiatry, 127,* 1391–1394. http://dx.doi.org/10.1176/ajp.127.10.1391.

Lindemann, E. (1944). Symptomatology and management of acute grief. *American Journal of Psychiatry, 101,* 141–148. http://dx.doi.org/10.1176/ajp .101.2.141.

Parad, L. G., & Parad, H. J. (1968). A study of crisis-oriented planned short-term treatment: Part II. *Social Casework, 49,* 418–426. http://dx.doi.org /10.1177/104438946804900705.

Rapoport, L. (1965). The state of crisis: Some theoretical considerations. In H. Parad (Ed.), *Crisis intervention: Selected readings* (pp. 22–31). New York, NY: Family Service Association of America.

Regel, S. (2007). Post-trauma support in the workplace: The current status and practice of critical incident stress management (CISM) and psychological debriefing (PD) with organizations in the UK. *Occupational Medicine, 57,* 411–416. http://dx.doi.org/10.1093/occmed/kqm071.

Regel, S., & Dyregrov, A. (2012). Commonalities and new directions in post-trauma support programs. In R. Hughes, A. Kinder, & C. Cooper (Eds.), *International handbook of workplace trauma and support* (pp. 48–67). New York, NY: Wiley.

Rose, S. C., Bisson, J., Churchill, R., & Wessely, S. (2002). Psychological debriefing for preventing post-traumatic stress disorder (PTSD). *Cochrane Database of Systematic Reviews* Issue 2. Art. No. CD000560. http://doi.org /10.1002/14651858.CD000560.

Salmon, T. (1919). War neuroses and their lesson. *New York Medical Journal, 108*, 993–994.

Seligman, M. E. P. (1995). The effectiveness of psychotherapy: The *Consumer Reports* study. *American Psychologist, 50*, 965–974. https://doi.org/10.1037 /0003-066X.50.12.965.

Solomon, Z., & Benbenishty, R. (1986). The role of proximity, immediacy, and expectancy in frontline treatment of combat stress reaction among Israelis in the Lebanon War. *American Journal of Psychiatry, 143*, 613–617.

Solomon, Z., Shklar, R., & Mikulincer, M. (2005). Frontline treatment of combat stress reaction: A 20-year longitudinal evaluation study. *American Journal of Psychiatry, 162*, 2309–2314.

Swanson, W. C., & Carbon, J. B. (1989). Crisis intervention: Theory and technique (Task Force Report of American Psychiatric Association). *Treatments of psychiatric disorders* (pp. 2520–2531). Washington, DC: APA Press.

Tamrakar, T., Murphy, J., & Elklit, A. (2019). Was debriefing dismissed too quickly? Assessment of the 2002 Cochrane review. *Crisis, Stress, and Human Resilience, 1*, 46–55.

Tuckey, M. R. (2007). Issues in the debriefing debate for the emergency services: Moving research outcomes forward. *Clinical Psychology Science and Practice, 14*, 106–116. http://dx.doi.org/10.1111/j.1468-2850.2007.00069.x.

Tuckey, M. R., & Scott, J. E. (2014). Group critical incident stress debriefing with emergency services personnel: A randomized controlled trial. *Anxiety, Stress, and Coping, 27*, 38–54. http://dx.doi.org/10.1080/10615806 .2013.809421.

United Nations (2020). *Policy brief: COVID-19 and the need for action on mental health.* Geneva, Switzerland: United Nations. https://www.un.org/sites /un2.un.org/files/un_policy_brief-covid_and_mental_health_final.pdf.

TWO | Structure and Mechanisms of Psychological First Aid

THE WORLD HEALTH ORGANIZATION (2010) has concluded that, in general, the demand for mental health services worldwide far exceeds the availability of mental health resources. This "gap" between demand and availability widens during mental health emergencies at the local level and disasters on the larger scale. When confronted with mental health challenges from disasters such as COVID-19, the United Nations recommends ensuring the widespread availability of emergency mental health / crisis intervention services not only to health care workers, emergency services personnel, and other frontline workers but in a "whole-society" continuum of care approach. "Mental health and psychosocial support must be available in any emergency" (United Nations, 2020, p. 3). They further recommend "building human resource capacity to deliver mental health and social care, for example among community workers so that they can provide support" (p. 4). To do this, new delivery paradigms must be utilized. Psychological first aid is one such paradigm. In a recent article in *Scientific American*, RAPID PFA training, based upon the model in this book, has been recommended for everyone (Editors, 2021). Let's take a closer look.

PFA

Integrating the two concepts of physical first aid and psychological crisis intervention mentioned in the previous chapter, *psychological first aid* (PFA) was born. The first noteworthy mention of PFA was in the context of a curriculum developed in 1944 for the United States Merchant Marine during World War II. The paper was read at the Centenary Meeting of the American Psychiatric Association in Philadelphia on May 15–18, 1944. Ironically, Lindemann introduced his work after the Cocoanut Grove Fire of 1942 (see chapter 1) at the same meeting. The Merchant Marine paper was later published in the *American Journal of Psychiatry* (Blain, Hoch, & Ryan, 1945). The authors noted, "Natural defense mechanisms such as fatalistic attitudes and wishful thinking lose their protective ability as the law of averages make each succeeding attack seem more dangerous to the individual. Can it be said that the strongest defense consists in the most active offense in the battle of nerves as it does in other battles? That here, also, fore-warning is fore-arming" (p. 629). Moreover, they noted, "Our suggested course in psychological first aid and prevention ... aims to help prevent the development of maladjustments and neurotic symptoms, and to aid people in dealing with their tensions and personal problems" (p. 631). The curriculum was developed to acknowledge that psychological distress on shipboard was a significant risk factor for poor performance and the development of psychological "casualties" at sea, especially during wartime.

The program consisted of seven topics:

1. What are war nerves?
2. Symptoms: diagnosis, cause, treatment, and prognosis
3. Understanding physical reactions
4. Understanding emotional reactions
5. Personal hygiene
6. Managing one's own adverse reactions (stress management; self-help)
7. Managing adverse reactions in others

The roots of psychological first aid were further expanded within the community of mental health providers when Thorne (1952) recognized the potential to mitigate adverse psychological sequelae through psychological first aid techniques that assisted in the rapid recognition of, and appropriate intervention for, current acute psychological distress. Thorne's proposed interventions included (1) providing *reassurance* (regarding patients' fears and problems); (2) providing *suggestions* for action (to deal with psychological symptoms in need of urgent attention); (3) allowing *catharsis* (involving reflection and clarification of feelings); and (4) using *persuasion, advice,* and *other supportive methods* (to deal with acute situational challenges beyond the patients' resources). In Thorne's view, mental health practitioners who did not recognize or address acute psychological distress in this way were "not functioning at the highest levels of professional competency" (p. 210).

In 1954, the American Psychiatric Association published the monograph entitled *Psychological First Aid in Community Disasters.* That document defined and argued for the development of an acute mental health intervention referred to as "psychological first aid." This early exposition noted,

> In all disasters, whether they result from the forces of nature or from enemy attack, the people involved are subjected to stresses of a severity and quality not generally encountered.... It is vital for all disaster workers to have some familiarity with common patterns of reaction to unusual emotional stress and strain. These workers must also know the fundamental principles of coping most effectively with disturbed people. Although [these suggestions have] been stimulated by the current needs for civil defense against possible enemy action.... These principles are essential for those who are to help the victims of floods, fires, tornadoes, and other natural catastrophes. (American Psychiatric Association, 1954, p. 5)

This document delineated the constituents of PFA to consist of (1) the ability to recognize common (and one might assume uncommon) reactions post disaster; and (2) the fundamentals of assisting others in coping with challenging situations and managing stress. The document also emphasized that *all* disaster workers should be trained in PFA, not just mental health clinicians.

In the first disaster mental health text *When Disaster Strikes*, Beverley Raphael (1986) noted, "In the first hours after a disaster, at least 25% of the population may be stunned and dazed, apathetic and wandering—suffering from the disaster syndrome—especially if impact has been sudden and totally devastating.... At this point, psychological first aid and triage ... are necessary" (p. 257). This reference to PFA represented an important rejuvenation of the concept.

In 1992, expanding the work of the International Critical Incident Stress Foundation, the American Red Cross (ARC) fielded a truly bold disaster mental health initiative in which all major ARC chapters were to have the capacity to provide mental health care to disaster survivors. The challenge facing ARC state disaster mental health chairpersons (and I, GSE, was chair of Maryland's ARC disaster mental health initiative) was selecting the specific psychological/behavioral tactics to employ.

While the modern era saw the development of many models of PFA, initiatives from the Johns Hopkins Bloomberg School of Public Health were among the first to lead to the curriculum development for, and subsequent training of, professional and paraprofessional community personnel to deliver PFA as a means of enhancing psychological surge capacity and fostering community resilience. More specifically, disasters were seen as challenges to the nation's public health and therefore fell under the mandate to develop training programs that fostered the public health of the nation. This public health perspective recognized that in the wake of disaster three important dynamics would occur:

1. Mental health "casualties" would far outnumber physical casualties, depending upon the cause of the disaster.
2. Psychological distress, trauma, and suicidal ideation were potentially contagious.
3. A distinct shortage of mental health clinicians available to provide acute psychological services meant personnel outside of the mental health professions, especially public health professionals,

educators, and emergency services personnel, needed to be trained (Everly, Beaton, et al., 2008; McCabe, Everly, et al., 2014)

The Institute of Medicine (IOM; 2003) noted that psychological first aid can provide the ability to increase skills, knowledge, and effectiveness in maximizing health and resilience. In a postdisaster context, the IOM characterized psychological first aid as a skill for reducing cognitive distress and negative health behaviors through (1) education on normal psychological responses to trauma; (2) active listening skills; (3) self-care through adequate sleep, rest, and nutrition; and (4) an awareness of when to seek help from professional care providers.

The US Department of Health and Human Services (2004) subsequently compiled a list of "immediate mental health interventions" that includes psychological first aid. The international community has recognized and adopted psychological first aid guidelines as well. The Inter-Agency Standing Committee (IASC) was established in 1992 in response to the United Nation's General Assembly Resolution 46/182. The resolution established the IASC as the primary mechanism for facilitating interagency decision making in response to complex emergencies and natural disasters. In its guidelines for mental health response, the IASC specifically mentions PFA, noting that most people experiencing acute mental distress following exposure to extreme stress are "best supported without medication" and that "all aid workers, and especially health workers, should be able to provide very basic psychological first aid" (2007, pp. 118–119).

The International Federation of Red Cross and Red Crescent Societies (2003) published its training manual *Community-Based Psychological Support*, in which it described core elements of physical protection and psychological support. Thus, PFA enjoys virtually universal recommendation for implementation in the wake of trauma and disaster. But what is the basis for such broad-based recommendations? As noted in the previous chapter, in a report published by the World Health Organization, Bisson and Lewis (2009) identified 74 published papers purporting to discuss PFA. The authors were unable to find empirical data supporting the use of PFA post disaster or trauma:

In summary, there is an absence of direct evidence for the effectiveness of PFA, but indirect evidence supports the delivery of services based on the principles of PFA in the first few weeks after a traumatic event. We agree that when delivered PFA should be consistent with research evidence on risk and resilience following trauma; applicable and practical in field settings; appropriate for developmental levels across the lifespan; and culturally informed and delivered in a flexible manner. (Bisson & Lewis, 2009, p. 15)

At the request of the Advisory Council of the American Red Cross Disaster Services, Fox et al. (2013) performed an independent comprehensive review of the effectiveness of PFA from 1990 through 2010. The goal was to assess the extant literature to determine whether PFA could be effectively provided by those without professional mental health training in the wake of disasters and potentially traumatic events. The authors identified 58 sources. Unfortunately, there were no controlled studies identified. After a thorough review of existing evidence, the authors concluded, "Sufficient evidence for psychological first aid is widely supported by available objective observations and expert opinion and best fits the category of 'evidence informed' but without proof of effectiveness. An intervention provided by volunteers without professional mental health training for people who have experienced a traumatic event offers an acceptable option. Further outcome research is recommended" (p. 247).

Core Concepts and Mechanisms of Action

So, what are the *core competencies* of PFA? Has there emerged a general consensus as to its tactical constituency? PFA is not the practice of medicine, clinical psychology, or social work, per se. It does not entail diagnosis or treatment. It is a form of psychological crisis intervention. Anyone who would typically be taught physical first aid can be taught psychological first aid. Therefore, consistent with historical precedents, it was accepted that non–mental health personnel should be trained to deliver psychological first aid. Public health workers, clergy, educators, law enforcement personnel, firefighters, emergency medical technicians, and military personnel have been identified as high priority target groups to receive training in PFA. These personnel are often referred to as "peer" interventionists.

PFA is a subset, or variation on the theme, of psychological crisis intervention. PFA may be considered the earliest point on the psychological continuum of care. According to the Institute of Medicine (2003, p. 7), "Psychological first aid is a group of skills identified to limit distress and negative health behaviors.... PFA generally includes education about normal psychological responses to stressful and traumatic events; skills in active listening; understanding the importance of maintaining physical health and normal sleep, nutrition, and rest; and understanding when to seek help from professional caregivers."

In her seminal clinical treatise, Raphael (1986) suggests that psychological first aid consists of the following:

1. Comfort and consolation
2. Physical protection
3. Provision of physical necessities
4. Channeling energy into constructive behaviors
5. Reuniting victims with friends, family
6. Provision of behavioral and/or emotional support, especially during emotionally taxing tasks
7. Allowing emotional ventilation
8. Reestablishing a sense of security
9. Utilization of acute social and community support networks
10. Triage and referral for those in acute need
11. Referral to subacute and ongoing support networks

Everly and Flynn (2006) attempted to provide further guidance into the nature of PFA by defining PFA and listing core behavioral elements:

1. Assessment of need for intervention (Level 1 assessment) — Note that the present use of the term *assessment* is not intended to refer to formal mental health assessment per se, rather, it is designed to refer more to an appraisal of functional psychological and behavioral status.

2. Stabilize—Subsequent to an initial assessment and determination that intervention of some form is warranted, act to prevent or reduce a worsening of the current psychological or behavioral status.

3. Assess and triage (Level 2 assessment)—Once initial stabilization has been achieved, further assessment is indicated with triage as a viable option. Assessment of functionality is the most essential aspect of this phase.

4. Communicate—Communicate concern, reassurance, and information regarding stress management.

5. Connect—Connect the person in distress to informal and/or formal support systems, if indicated.

The National Institute of Mental Health document *Mental Health and Mass Violence* (2002) has enumerated the functions of psychological first aid as including the need to

- protect survivors from further harm,
- reduce physiological arousal,
- mobilize support for those who are most distressed,
- keep families together and facilitate reunions with loved ones,
- provide information and foster communication and education, and
- use effective risk communication techniques. (p. 13)

The IASC, in its guidelines for mental health response, specifically mentions PFA and enumerates it as follows:

PFA is often mistakenly seen as a clinical or emergency psychiatric intervention. Rather, it is a description of a humane, supportive response to a fellow human being who is suffering and who may need support. PFA encompasses:

1. Protecting from further harm (in rare situations, very distressed persons may take decisions that put them at further risk of harm). Where appropriate, inform distressed survivors of their right to refuse to discuss the events with (other) aid workers or with journalists.

2. Providing the opportunity for survivors to talk about the events, but without pressure. Respect the wish not to talk and avoid pushing for more information than the person may be ready to give.

3. Listening patiently in an accepting and non-judgmental manner.

4. Conveying genuine compassion.

5. Identifying basic practical needs and ensuring that these are met.

6. Asking for people's concerns and trying to address these.

7. Discouraging negative ways of coping (specifically discouraging coping through use of alcohol and other substances, explaining that people in severe distress are at much higher risk of developing substance use problems).

8. Encouraging participation in normal daily routines (if possible) and use of positive means of coping (e.g., culturally appropriate relaxation methods, accessing helpful cultural and spiritual supports).

9. Encouraging, but not forcing, company from one or more family member or friends.

10. As appropriate, offering the possibility to return for further support.

11. As appropriate, referring to locally available support mechanisms or to trained clinicians. (IASC, 2007, pp. 119–20)

Hobfoll et al. (2007) distilled previous definitions of psychological first aid into five generic intervention principles/goals: (1) establish a sense of safety; (2) calm; (3) instill a sense of being able to solve problems for oneself or as part of a group (such as family, school, religious, or community group); (4) establish social support; and (5) foster hope.

Everly, Beaton, et al. (2008) reported the Centers for Disease Control and Prevention (CDC) / Association of Schools and Programs of Public Health (ASPPH) recommendations for the core competencies in disaster mental health. In 2000, the CDC and ASPPH established the Centers for Public Health Preparedness (CPHP) to educate and train the public health workforce to prepare and respond to acts of domestic terrorism, as well as other disasters that might threaten the public health and welfare of the United States. In 2004, CDC and ASPPH directed CPHP network members to create the CPHP Mental Health and Psychosocial Preparedness Exemplar Group to address the mental health aspects of terrorism and mass disasters. The CPHP Mental Health and Psychosocial Preparedness Exemplar Group transitioned into the Disaster Mental Health Collaborative Group in 2006. The resulting consensus document containing five core competencies in disaster mental health begins:

> The following represents the consensus core competencies for disaster mental, psychosocial, and behavioral health preparedness and response. These competencies can serve as a framework for the development of training programs, educational curricula, evaluation processes, and organizational and human development initiatives, such as job descriptions and performance evaluations. These competencies must be integrated within organizational structure and incident management systems and are guided by the following principles [of] adherence to performance within one's scope of practice … consideration of the context of the situation … sensitivity to diversity and cultural competence … recognition of the desire to reduce the risk of any harm that may come from intervention [and] recognition of the importance of teamwork and adherence to the incident command system. (pp. 540–541)

In addition, the Collaborative Group's recommendations stated that disaster response personnel will demonstrate the ability to communicate effectively, assess the need for and type of intervention (if any), develop and implement an action plan (based on one's knowledge, skill, authority, and functional role) to meet those needs identified through assessment, and care for responder peers and self.

More expert consensus recommendations are those of McCabe, Everly, et al. (2014) who reported on the development of a consensus-derived, empirically supported, competency-based PFA training model. The project was conducted as part of a larger effort by 14 CDC-funded Preparedness and Emergency Response Learning Centers in accredited schools of public health. The PFA training model uniquely offers a knowledge, skills, and attitudes (KSA) approach to content for each of the PFA competency statements in the model. The resulting product consists of an 18-cell matrix of consensus-based empirically supported KSAs constituting six PFA competency domains: (1) initial contact, rapport building, and stabilization; (2) brief assessment and triage; (3) intervention; (4) triage; (5) referral, liaison, and advocacy; and (6) self-awareness and self-care.

What, then, are the distilled core components, or competencies, of PFA? Although these factors may be discussed, if not debated, as in any developing field, it is nevertheless believed that PFA consists of a set of core competencies:

1. Stabilization—interventions designed to stop escalating psychological and behavioral reactions, discourage impulsive actions, and instill a sense of calm.

2. Assessment—the determination of current psychological and behavioral status especially with regard to one's ability to function in a constructive manner and attend to one's basic responsibilities to self and others (i.e., the determination of the need for crisis intervention).

3. Psychological triage (prioritization)—determination of the urgency of need for intervention.

4 Supportive communications—the ability to communicate in a manner that shows respect, compassion, and concern and that fosters continued dialogue and compliance, if indicated.

5. Acute interventions—psychological and behavioral interventions designed to mitigate acute distress and instill hope, such as anticipatory guidance (setting expectations), explanatory guidance (explaining current reactions), and even prescriptive guidance, such as stress management and cognitive reframing.

6. Facilitation of access to continued support or care (skills in liaison and advocacy), if indicated.

7. Practice of buddy care and self-care for interventionists.

Validation of the Johns Hopkins Rapid PFA Model

The Johns Hopkins RAPID PFA model is unique in that it is historically based, theory driven, evidence informed, and evidenced based. The development and validation of the model was guided by the assertions of Harvard psychiatry professor Theodore Millon who argued that the construction of an effective clinical science requires a historical review, a firm theoretical base, as well as indirect (evidence-informed) and direct (evidence-based) validation (Millon, 1987). While our own work described in the preface and the guidelines reviewed in previous sections of this chapter and the previous chapter provided a foundation of expert opinion for the construction of a platform for PFA, we sought theoretical grounding as well. To answer the question of how PFA should be instrumentally structured to yield the most effective clinical outcome, we reviewed seminal work in the area of human stress, stress management, and human resilience. The postulations of Selye, the clinical formulations of Beck and Lazarus and Folkman, as well as the integrative work of Everly, served as the theoretical underpinnings of the extant model (see Everly & Lating, 2019, for a thorough review). Various expert consensus reports supported by the CDC, ASPPH, and other organizations also served to shape the extant model (Everly, Beaton, et al., 2008; Everly, Hamilton, et al., 2008; Everly, Perrin, & Everly, 2008; Hoffman et al., 2005; McCabe, Everly, et al., 2014; Sheehan, Everly, & Langlieb, 2004).

Having identified historical and theoretical platforms, we sought empirical validation for essential components of the model. Relying upon our own structural modeling research spanning 20 years (Smith et al., 2020; Smith, Everly, & Haight, 2012), we refined the componential infrastructure using repeated structured equation modeling. We followed that by conducting content validation studies using more than 1,500 participants and found that RAPID PFA training led to improvements in participant knowledge, confidence, and preparedness for applying PFA as well as personal resilience, which supports the notion that knowledge engenders resilience-related self-efficacy (Everly et al., 2014; Everly & Kennedy, 2019). In another series of investigations, we found that our training model with preparedness components added increased personal preparedness knowledge and attitudes in addition to increased community preparedness and resilience planning (McCabe, Semon, et al., 2014). More recently, a randomized cohort design found that nurses who received RAPID PFA training reported enhanced disaster preparedness, increased self-efficacy, and positive attitudes regarding the use of PFA (Said, 2021).

In a relatively small randomized clinical trial, we also discovered that RAPID PFA was associated with a decline in acute distress compared to a cathartic ventilation process alone (Everly et al., 2016). As a natural corollary to that research, we tested the ability of the core PFA protocol to reduce acute distress when applied in a group format (Despeaux et al., 2019). Results of that study confirmed the ability of the PFA model to not only reduce acute distress but to be superior when compared to another model of PFA whose active mechanisms consisted of cathartic ventilation and referral alone (sometimes termed a "listen and refer" model of PFA). Finally, we conducted a longitudinal study of the effects of the basic training curriculum itself. While we had sufficient data on the concurrent content validation of two variations of the curriculum and ability of the curriculum to improve acute perceptions of resilience, we were interested in the ability of the core curriculum to exert a lasting effect. Noullet et al. (2018) found participating in the core PFA curriculum appeared to increase resilience and exert a protective effect against burnout and vicarious trauma lasting at least 12 months. This finding is in concert with the findings of Solomon reported in chapter 1.

COVID-19 Implications for the Implementation of the Rapid PFA Model

We have described that psychological first aid is an analogue to physical first aid. The COVID-19 pandemic, which will be described in more detail in subsequent chapters, has caused a necessary shift in reliance on telemedicine, which has typically utilized telephonic and "virtual" video-based internet platforms (Grady et al., 2011). A natural question to arise is whether PFA can be provided in this forum. In our opinion, the answer is an emphatic yes. Telephone crisis hotlines have functioned effectively for more than 70 years, so performing virtual PFA, which utilizes audio and visual images, provides substantial advantages over voice communication alone. The use of virtual PFA is predicated on the assumptions that these services can be provided securely and reliably. For example, questionable security and internet glitches and outages will clearly hinder the effective provision of these services.

KEY POINT SUMMARY

1. Psychological first aid (PFA) may be defined as a supportive and compassionate presence designed to first stabilize, then mitigate acute distress, and finally facilitate access to continued care, if indicated. It is applicable to a wide variety of target groups, including health care professionals (Everly, 2020a), community members (Everly, 2020b), veterinarians (Nusbaum, Wenzel, Everly, 2007), nurses (Everly et al., 2010), the faith-based community (McCabe et al., 2008), and emergency service and disaster response professionals, including law enforcement (Castellano, 2018; Sheehan, Everly, & Langlieb, 2004).

2. PFA has almost universal endorsement by national and international agencies; however, its recommendations are based primarily upon expert opinion and evidence-informed research.

3. There is a constellation of core active ingredients within PFA consisting of stabilization, assessment, triage, acute intervention for mitigation of distress, and referral/liaison/advocacy.

4. The Johns Hopkins RAPID PFA model is unique in that it is theory-driven, evidence- informed, and empirically validated. The PFA model and its core active mechanisms have shown the ability to reduce acute distress when delivered in individual and group formats. The curriculum has not only shown content validity but appears to enhance perceptions of personal resilience and potentially exert a protective effect against burnout and vicarious trauma supporting the notion that knowledge engenders self-efficacy and personal

resilience. Finally, the curriculum, which can be delivered in telephonic or virtual formats, also seems to contribute to community public health preparedness when combined with a community-planning component.

5. Self-care and buddy care should be considered essential elements of PFA.

References

American Psychiatric Association. (1954). *Psychological first aid in community disasters*. Washington, DC: American Psychiatric Association.

Bisson, J. I., & Lewis, C. (2009). *Systematic review of psychological first aid*. Commissioned by the World Health Organization. Geneva, Switzerland: World Health Organization.

Blain, D., Hoch, P., & Ryan, V. G. (1945). A course in psychological first aid and prevention. *American Journal of Psychiatry, 101*, 629–634. http://dx.doi.org/10.1176/ajp.101.5.629.

Castellano, C. (2018). Silver award: Reciprocal peer support for addressing mental health crises among police, veterans, mothers of special needs children, and others. 2018 APA Psychiatric Services Achievement Awards. *Psychiatric Services, 69*, e7–8. http://dx.doi.org/10.1176/appi.ps.691006.

Despeaux, K. E., Lating, J. M., Everly, G. S., Jr., Sherman, M. F., & Kirkhart, M. W. (2019). A randomized controlled trial assessing the efficacy of group psychological first aid. *Journal of Nervous and Mental Disease, 207*, 626–632. http://dx.doi.org/10.1097/NMD.0000000000001029.

Editors. (2021, February). A step to ease the pandemic mental health crisis. *Scientific American, 324*, 10. http://doi.org/10.1038/scientificamerican0221-10.

Eisdorpher, C., & Golann, S. (1969). Principles for the training of "new professionals" in mental health. *Community Mental Health Journal, 5*, 349–357. http://dx.doi.org/10.1007/BF01438980.

Everly, G. S., Jr. (2020a). Psychological first aid to support healthcare professionals. *Journal of Patient Safety and Risk Management, 25*, 159–162. https://doi.org/10.1177/2516043520944637.

Everly, G. S., Jr. (2020b). Psychological first aid (PFA) to expand mental health support and foster resiliency in underserved and access-compromised areas. *Crisis, Stress, and Human Resilience, 1*, 227–232.

Everly, G. S., Jr., Barnett, D. B., Sperry, N., & Links, J. M. (2010). The use of psychological first aid (PFA) training among nurses to enhance population resiliency. *International Journal of Emergency Mental Health, 12*, 21–30.

Everly, G. S., Jr., Beaton, R. D., Pfefferbaum, B., & Parker, C. L. (2008). Training for disaster response personnel: The development of proposed core competencies in disaster mental health. *Public Health Reports, 123,* 13–19.

Everly, G. S., Jr., & Flynn, B. (2006). Principles and practical procedures for acute psychological first aid training for personnel without mental health experience. *International Journal of Emergency Mental Health, 8,* 93–100.

Everly, G. S., Jr., Hamilton, S. E., Tyiska, C. G., & Ellers, K. (2008). Mental health response to disaster: Consensus recommendations: Early Psychological Intervention Subcommittee (EPI), National Volunteer Organizations Active in Disaster (NVOAD). *Aggression and Violent Behavior, 13,* 407–412.

Everly, G. S., Jr., & Kennedy, C. (2019). Content validation of the Johns Hopkins model of psychological first Aid (RAPID-PFA) expanded curriculum. *Crisis, Stress, and Human Resilience, 1,* 6–14.

Everly, G. S., Jr., Lating, J. M., Sherman, M., & Goncher, I. (2016). The potential efficacy of psychological first aid on self-reported anxiety and mood: A pilot study. *Journal of Nervous and Mental Disease, 204,* 233–235. http://dx .doi.org/10.1097/NMD.0000000000000429.

Everly, G. S., Jr., McCabe, O. L., Semon, N., Thompson, C. B., & Links, J. (2014). The development of a model of psychological first aid for non–mental health trained public health personnel: The Johns Hopkins RAPID-PFA. *Journal of Public Health Management and Practice, 20,* S24–S29. http://dx.doi .org/10.1097/PHH.0000000000000065.

Everly, G. S., Jr., Perrin, P., & Everly, G. S., III. (2008). Psychological issues in escape, recovery, and survival in the wake of disaster. *Monograph released by the National Institute of Occupational Safety and Health (NIOSH), Pittsburgh Research Laboratory.*

Fox, J. H., Burkle, F. M., Jr., Bass, J., Pia, F. A., Epstein, J. L., & Markenson, D. (2013). The effectiveness of psychological first aid as a disaster intervention tool: Research analysis of peer-reviewed literature from 1990–2010. *Disaster Medicine and Public Health Preparedness, 6,* 247–252. http://dx .doi.org/10.1001/dmp.2012.39.

Grady, B., Myers, K. M., Nelson, E-L., Belz, N., Bennett, L., Carnahan, L., . . . Voyles, D. (2011). Evidence-based practice for telemental health. *Telemedicine and e-Health, 17.* http://dx.doi.org/10.1089/tmj.2010.0158.

Hobfoll, S. E., Watson, P., Bell, C. C., Bryant, R. A., Brymer, M. J., Friedman, M. J., . . . Ursano, R. J. (2007). Five essential elements of immediate and mid-term mass trauma intervention: Empirical evidence. *Psychiatry, 70,* 283–315. http://dx.doi.org/10.1521/psyc.2007.70.4.283.

Hoffman, Y., Everly, G. S., Jr., Werner, D., Livet, M., Madrid, P. A., Pfefferbaum, B., & Beaton, R. (2005). Identification and evaluation of mental health and psychosocial preparedness resources from the Centers for Public Health Preparedness. *Journal of Public Health Management and Practice, 11*(6 Suppl), S138–S142.

Institute of Medicine. (2003). *Preparing for the psychological consequences of terrorism: A public health strategy.* Washington, DC: National Academy of Sciences.

International Federation of Red Cross and Red Crescent Societies. (2003). *Community-based psychological support: A training manual.* Geneva, Switzerland: International Federation of Red Cross.

Inter-Agency Standing Committee. (2007). *IASC guidelines on mental health and psychosocial support in emergency settings.* Geneva, Switzerland: IASC.

McCabe, O. L., Everly, G. S., Jr., Brown, L. M., Wendelboe, A. M., Abd Hamid, N. H., Tallchief, V. L., & Links, J. M. (2014). Psychological first aid: A consensus-derived, empirically supported, competency-based training model. *American Journal of Public Health, 104,* 621–628. http://dx.doi.org/10.2105/AJPH.2013.301219.

McCabe, O. L., Lating, J. M., Everly, G. S., Jr., Mosley, A., Teague, P., Links, J., & Kaminsky, M. J. (2008). Psychological first aid training for the faith community: A model curriculum. *International Journal of Emergency Mental Health, 9,* 181–192.

McCabe, O. L., Semon, N. L., Thompson, C. B., Lating, J. M., Everly, G. S., Jr., Perry, C. J., … Links, J. M. (2014). Building a national model of public mental health preparedness and community resilience: Validation of a dual-intervention, systems-based approach. *Disaster Medicine and Public Health Preparedness, 8,* 511–526. http://dx.doi.org/10.1017/dmp.2014.119.

Millon, T. (1987). *Manual for the MCMI-II.* Minneapolis, MN: National Computer Systems.

National Institute of Mental Health. (2002). *Mental health and mass violence: Evidence-based early psychological intervention for victims/survivors of mass violence: A workshop to reach consensus on best practices.* (NIH Publication No. 02-5138). Washington, DC: National Institute of Mental Health.

Noullet, C., Lating, J. M., Kirkhart, M. W., Dewey, R., & Everly, G. S., Jr. (2018). Effects of pastoral crisis intervention training on resilience and compassion fatigue in clergy: A pilot study. *Spirituality in Clinical Practice, 5,* 1–7. http://dx.doi.org/10.1037/scp0000158.

Nusbaum, K. E., Wenzel, J. G. W., & Everly, G. S., Jr. (2007). Psychological first aid and veterinarians in rural communities undergoing livestock depopulation. *Journal of the American Veterinary Medical Association, 231,* 692–694. http://dx.doi.org/10.2460/javma.231.5.692.

Raphael, B. (1986). *When disaster strikes: How individuals and communities cope with catastrophe.* New York, NY: Basic Books.

Said, N. (2021). *Psychological first aid training for disaster preparedness in nurses: A non-equivalent control group study* [Doctoral dissertation, An-Najah National University]. PolyU Electronic Theses, https://theses.lib.polyu.edu.hk/handle/200/11160.

Sheehan, D., Everly, G. S., Jr., & Langlieb, A. (2004). Current best practices coping with major critical incidents. *FBI Law Enforcement Bulletin, 73,* 1–13.

Smith, K. J., Emerson, D. J., Boster, C. R., & Everly, G. S., Jr. (2020). Resilience as a coping strategy for reducing auditor turnover intentions. Accounting Research Journal, *33,* 483–498. http://dx.doi.org/10.1108/ARJ-09-2019-0177.

Smith, K. J., Everly, G. S., Jr., Haight, G. T. (2012). SAS4: Validation of a four-item measure of worry and rumination. *Advances in Accounting Behavioral Research, 15,* 101–131. http://dx.doi.org/10.1108/S1475-1488(2012)0000015 009.

Thorne, F. C. (1952). Psychological first aid. *Journal of Clinical Psychology, 8,* 210–211.

Tuckey, M. R. (2007). Issues in the debriefing debate for the emergency services: Moving research outcomes forward. *Clinical Psychology Science and Practice, 14,* 106–116. http://dx.doi.org/10.1111/j.1468-2850.2007.00069.x.

United Nations (2020). *Policy brief: COVID-19 and the need for action on mental health.* Geneva, Switzerland: United Nations. https://www.un.org/sites/un2.un.org/files/un_policy_brief-covid_and_mental_health_final.pdf.

United States Department of Health and Human Services. (2004). *Mental health response to mass violence and terrorism* (DHHS No. SMA 3959). Rockville, MD: Center for Mental Health Services, SAMHSA.

World Health Organization (2010). *mhGAP Intervention Guide.* Geneva, Switzerland: World Health Organization.

THREE | Psychological Consequences of Trauma

What You Will Encounter in the Field

IN CHAPTERS 1 AND 2, WE DEFINED psychological first aid (PFA), provided a brief developmental history, and discussed its structure and mechanisms of action. Now we will focus on common psychological and behavioral reactions that reside in the wake of trauma and disaster. This discussion should begin to set expectations for the challenges you will face implementing PFA. Similarly, a rationale will emerge for promoting the implementation and proliferation of PFA currently and in the future.

Traumatic incidents and disasters are adverse events embedded in the fabric of human history, and their physical and emotional consequences may be varied and profound. The attacks of September 11, 2001, the tsunami in South and Southeast Asia in December 2004, Hurricane Katrina in August 2005, the shootings at Virginia Tech in April 2007, the earthquake in Haiti in 2010, the *Deepwater Horizon* disaster in 2010, the Boston Marathon bombings in April 2013, the terrorist attacks in Paris in 2015 and in Jakarta in 2016, and the COVID-19 pandemic that began in December 2019 are just some examples of the ubiquitous nature of disasters.

While large-scale disasters and community-wide emergencies, such as in Ferguson, Missouri; Charleston, South Carolina; Paris, France; Orlando, Florida; and Minneapolis, Minnesota, typically garner national and international attention, daily smaller-scale traumatic events, such as shootings, assaults, floods, fires, and accidents, are equally as impactful for those who experience them. What these incidents seem to share in common "is their potential to affect many persons simultaneously and to engender an array of psychological stressors, including threat to one's own life and physical integrity, exposure to the dead and dying, bereavement, profound loss, social and community disruption, and ongoing hardship" (Norris et al., 2002, p. 207). Ogle, Rubin, Berntsen, and Siegler (2013) reported that approximately 90% of the US population will be exposed to one or more traumatic events during their lifetime.

The majority of survivors of extreme adversity are normal people experiencing extraordinary circumstances who are typically able to function reasonably well. Moreover, there is growing recognition that many, if not most, people exposed to traumatic events are resilient and do not experience serious protracted disruptions in normal life functioning following a traumatic event (Bonanno, 2004; Bonanno et al., 2010; Mancini & Bonanno, 2006). However, while overall life functioning is quickly recovered in resilient people, PFA might be a contributing factor in maintaining or enhancing resilience in those who do not possess intrinsic resilience-promoting characteristics (American Psychiatric Association, 1954; Everly, 2013; Ruzek et al., 2007).

There are myriad adverse responses and consequences that you might encounter in the wake of adversity. The preponderance of studies assessing the emotional impact of disasters and traumatic events has focused on six reactions. Familiarity with the nature and prevalence of these reactions is advisable for anyone practicing PFA. We shall review (1) posttraumatic stress disorder, or PTSD; (2) depression; (3) anxiety; (4) panic disorder; (5) substance use disorders in survivors of disasters and traumatic events; and (6) psychophysiological stress reactions.

Although we have chosen to focus on these six relatively common or especially relevant syndromes, the information provided in this chapter is meant to familiarize those who intend to apply PFA to survivors who might manifest the symptoms and characteristics of these disorders and reactions commonly experienced following adverse events. It is not meant to be a diagnostic compendium. As you review the general characteristics of these disorders and reactions, it is important to recognize that some symptoms are normal responses to extreme adversity; thus, a responder providing PFA should not assume that a survivor has a disorder, or requires additional treatment, solely because he is experiencing or reporting *some* of these symptoms. Rather, each survivor's presenting symptoms and level of impairment should be evaluated, not on whether the person satisfies the criteria used for diagnosis but, rather, always on an individual basis and considered with regard to how any or all of the presenting signs and symptoms affect the person, specifically with regard to the degree of functional impairment and interference with necessary activities of current life. This point is key. In addition, and as will be addressed in more depth in chapter 13, PFA responders are often exposed to the effects of traumatic events, so they also should be considered at vicarious risk for some symptoms associated with the following disorders and reactions.

Posttraumatic Stress Disorder

There has been much media attention to posttraumatic stress disorder (PTSD), especially after the wars in the Middle East, and more recently the COVID-19 pandemic. The *DSM-5* (*Diagnostic and Statistical Manual of Mental Disorders*, fifth edition), which in the United States serves as the universal authority for psychiatric diagnosis, classifies PTSD as a trauma- and stressor-related disorder. Although the clinical presentations will vary, the hallmark of PTSD is exposure (either directly, witnessing, learning of the event, or repeated exposure to aversive event details, such as first responders excavating bodies) to at least one traumatic event (e.g., actual or threatened death, serious injury, sexual violence, torture) and the occurrence of symptoms after exposure to the event. PTSD symptoms must cause distress *and* dysfunction and are organized into the following four criteria:

1. Experiencing intrusive symptoms (e.g., distressing dreams, intrusive flashbacks).
2. Avoiding, often deliberately, stimuli associated with the event (e.g., thoughts, feelings, people, places).
3. Developing negative alterations in cognitions and mood (memory difficulties, exaggerated negative personal beliefs, fear, guilt, decreased interest in activities, and an inability to feel positive emotions).
4. Developing altered arousal (e.g., exaggerated startle response, quick tempered, hypervigilance, decreased concentration, sleep difficulties). (American Psychiatric Association, 2013)

Symptoms typically develop within the first three months of the trauma, need to be present for more than one month, and cause distressed or impaired functioning (American Psychiatric Association, 2013).

The estimated lifetime prevalence rate of PTSD in the United States is 8.7% (Kessler et al., 2005), with lower estimates occurring at around 0.5% to 1.0% in Europe, Asia, Africa, and Latin America (Hinton & Lewis-Fernández, 2011). In a large systematic literature review of US, Canadian, and UK military personnel serving in Iraq and Afghanistan, rates of PTSD were estimated to be 13.2% for those in the army, 10.4% for those in the marines, and 7.3% for those in the navy (Hines et al., 2014). PTSD rates for firefighters have been reported to range from 4.2% (Meyer et al., 2012) to as high as 37% (Bryant & Harvey, 1995). PTSD rates for police officers have been reported to be around 6% to 8% (Hartley et al., 2013; Martin, Marchand, & Boyer, 2009). And for ambulance personnel, PTSD rates are reported to be around 20% (Bennett et al., 2005; Jonsson, Segesten, & Mattsson, 2003). From a national survey of more than 3,000 women, those with rape histories involving both substance facilitation and forcible tactics had prevalence of PTSD at 36% (Zinzow et al., 2012). Previous research has documented an inverse J-shaped recovery curve for PTSD after traumatic events, with recovery being most rapid in the first year, more gradual in the second year, and stabilizing into chronicity after two years (Kessler et al., 1995).

The diagnostic criteria of PTSD fail to reveal the most important aspect of the disorder, however. Why is it that only about 9% of people exposed to a traumatic event develop PTSD and 91% do not? What is the defining moment of a psychological trauma? According to Everly and Lating (2004), the defining moment of psychological traumatization is when some experience violates some deeply held belief or worldview. While some traumatic events, such as burns and traumatic brain injury, are pathophysiologic exceptions to this rule, when survivors discuss adverse experiences, the PFA interventionist should be listening for ways in which the event may have violated a deeply held core belief the survivors hold about themselves or the world. It will provide some understanding of the current condition as well as provide some insight into whether there is a subsequent need for psychotherapy.

Depression

When we think of depression, we typically think of sadness, but where does sadness end and depression begin? The *DSM-5* refers to clinical depression as major depressive disorder (MDD). MDD is defined by an unregulated mood that also entails symptoms resulting in clinically significant distress or impairment wherein an individual experiences five or more symptoms for at least two weeks. These symptoms represent a change from a previous level of functioning, and the symptoms are not attributable to another medical condition (American Psychiatric Association, 2013). These symptoms are

1. depressed mood most of the day,
2. diminished interest or pleasure in activities (i.e., anhedonia),
3. significant weight loss or weight gain,
4. insomnia or hypersomnia,
5. psychomotor agitation (e.g., pacing, inability to sit still) or retardation (e.g., slowed speech or movements),
6. fatigue or loss of energy,
7. feelings of worthlessness or excessive guilt,

8. diminished ability to concentrate or indecisiveness, or
9. reoccurring thoughts of death or suicidal ideation (American Psychiatric Association, 2013).

To receive an MDD diagnosis, the symptoms need to result in impairment in relevant areas of functioning (e.g., social, occupational). Many of the symptoms of depression can be considered normal reactions immediately after a disaster or traumatic event, so determining what is normal and what is pathologic can be difficult. For example, feelings of grief are likely to be present in those newly bereaved, so they might display all or most of the symptoms described. With the exception of active suicidal ideation, these symptoms would represent a normal grief reaction and are not likely to be considered pathological. However, if the person is *seriously* functionally impaired because of these symptoms, or if the symptoms worsen over time, then a mental health professional *should* be consulted or a referral made regardless of whether the reactions seem etiologically understandable.

Of interest to the field of disaster and trauma research, as well as to PFA providers, is the suggestion that 25% of depressive episodes might have an identifiable trigger (Kaplan & Sadock, 1996), something the affected person readily identifies as the cause of his or her current depressive episode. In the case of a disaster, the difficulties and stress of experiencing and surviving a traumatic event might be thought of as triggering the symptoms associated with depression.

In addition, the course and symptoms of MDD are quite variable, and when subsymptoms of the diagnostic criteria are considered, Fried and Neese (2015) reported 16,400 different combinations of profiles that qualify for a diagnosis of MDD. In their study investigating the unique symptom profiles reported by 3,703 depressed outpatients, Fried and Neese (2015) found that the most common symptom profile was endorsed by only 1.8% of participants, and 14% of the sample endorsed unique profiles not shared by anyone else in the study. Regarding the symptoms that comprise MDD, a mnemonic credited to Carey Gross often used in the field to assess MDD, and one that might be helpful for those administering PFA, is **SIG-E-CAPSS**, which corresponds to

S leep disturbance: insomnia or hypersomnia

I nterest in usual activities: decreased

G uilt: excessive

E nergy: reduced

C oncentration: decreased

A ppetite disturbance resulting in weight loss or gain

P sychomotor agitation or retardation

S adness in mood most every day

S uicidal thoughts that are recurrent

The 12-month prevalence of major depression, based on structured interview samples of the US population, is estimated to be 7%, with lifetime prevalence at about 16% (American Psychiatric Association, 2013; Kessler et al., 2003). Beginning in early adolescence, women in the United States experience 1.5 to 3 times higher rates of depression than do men (Kessler et al., 2003). Estimated to affect between 250 million and 350 million people worldwide, depression is considered the leading cause of worldwide disability (Marcus et al., 2012; World Health Organization, 2020). The estimated 12-month prevalence rates in nondisplaced international samples demonstrate considerable variability, ranging from 0.8% to 5.8% in different countries (American Psychiatric Association, 2013; Weissman et al., 1996). In addition, police officers have had estimated rates of depression ranging from 12.0% (Hartley et al., 2011) to 37.2% (Lawson, Rodwell, & Noblet, 2012), whereas ambulance personnel have been estimated to have clinical levels of depression at 9% (Bennett et al., 2005). Women with rape histories have a prevalence rate of major depressive episodes of 36% (Zinzow et al., 2012). In a one-year longitudinal study of 1,054 participants in Detroit, Michigan, those who experienced at least one traumatic event were 1.71 times more likely to have greater depression severity compared to those who did not experience a traumatic event (Tracy et al., 2014).

Generalized Anxiety

Anxiety is different from fear. This point is confusing. Fear is stimulus specific, causing arousal and apprehension—a fear of snakes, for example. Anxiety is generalized apprehension and arousal, free floating and less associated with a highly defined specific stimulus. *DSM-5* classifies general anxiety disorder (GAD) as a set of symptoms that result in clinically significant distress or impairment and includes excessive anxiety (anticipation of future threat) and worry (apprehensive expectation) that occur more days than not for six months about a potentially wide array of events or activities and results in difficulty controlling the worry (American Psychiatric Association, 2013). Anxiety and worry in adults are associated with at least three of the following symptoms being present (only one needs to be present for children): (1) restlessness, (2) being easily fatigued, (3) difficulty concentrating, (4) irritability, (5) muscle tension, or (6) sleep disturbance (difficulty falling or staying asleep or unsatisfying sleep) (American Psychiatric Association, 2013).

The 12-month prevalence of GAD in the US population is estimated to be 2.9% (American Psychiatric Association, 2013; Kessler et al., 2005). A diagnosis of GAD can be difficult to make because many of the symptoms overlap with other disorders, particularly with depression and PTSD. Many individuals live with low levels of these symptoms, which may be exacerbated following a disaster; thus, recognizing this disorder is an important part of a postdisaster assessment. If GAD is exaggerated because of a trauma or a disaster, it can be paralyzing and stifle adherence and personal recovery initiatives.

In nondisplaced samples from other countries (e.g., China, South Korea, Japan, South Africa, and Australia), 12-month GAD rates have been found to range from 0.4% to 3.6% but have been reported to be as low as 0.0% in Nigeria (Lewis-Fernández et al., 2010). In a sample of 1,423 refugees, the estimated rate of GAD was 4% (Fazel, Wheeler, & Danesh, 2005), while in a sample of 517 patients admitted to an emergency department in Israel with somatic complaints but no discernible physical disorder, the incidence of GAD was 2.7% (Klein et al., 2013). In a sample of motor vehicle accident victims with PTSD, 7.8% had a co-morbid diagnosis of GAD (Kupchik et al., 2007). In a study comparing 72 adults who lost their savings in a bank fraud with 66 matched controls, those who experienced the loss had a rate of GAD at 27% compared to 10% of those in the control group (Ganzini, McFarland, & Cutler, 1990).

Panic Disorder

Like fear, panic is often confused with anxiety. Anxious people can indeed have panic attacks, but panic disorder (recurrent disabling panic attacks) is the syndrome of apprehension and arousal that reaches a whole different level of intensity and clinical challenge. The DSM-5 describes panic disorder as recurrent unexpected (i.e., no obvious cues or triggers) panic attacks. A panic attack is an abrupt surge of intense arousal that reaches an apex within minutes and entails symptoms such as heart pounding, sweating, shaking, chest pain, nausea, and fear of dying. To receive a diagnosis of panic disorder, the panic attack, which is not a mental disorder, is accompanied for at least one month by either persistent worry about having additional attacks, maladaptive changes in behavior related to the attacks (e.g., avoidance of places or situations that might evoke an attack), or both; is not attributable to drugs or medications; and is not explained more parsimoniously by another diagnosis (e.g., social anxiety or a specific phobia). The 12-month estimated prevalence for panic disorder in the United States and in several European countries is about 2% to 3% in adults and adolescents, with lower rates for Asian, African, and Latin countries, at around 0.1% to 0.8% (American Psychiatric Association, 2013).

The prevalence in women outnumbers the prevalence in men 2:1 (American Psychiatric Association, 2013). Panic disorder is associated with psychiatric and physical comorbidity, suicidal ideation and attempts, and overall decreased quality of life (Bovasso & Eaton, 1999; Cramer, Torgersen, & Kringlen, 2005; Goodwin et al., 2001; Kinley et al., 2009; Sareen et al., 2005). In a representative sample of 4,181 German participants, panic disorder was significantly associated with cardiovascular diseases and peripheral vascular disease (Tully & Baune, 2014). In a population-based sample of 8,441 active Canadian military personnel, results revealed that panic disorder and panic attacks occurred at a prevalence rate of 1.8% and 7.0%, respectively, and both were related to suicidal ideation and emotional distress (Kinley et al., 2011). In a 12-month longitudinal study of 1,589 residents that assessed peri-event panic attacks (i.e., a panic attack that occurs during or shortly after exposure to a traumatic event) and panic disorder following the March 11, 2004, train bombing in Madrid, in which 10 explosions killed 191 people and injured more than 2,000 others, the results revealed that the prevalence of peri-event panic attacks was 10.9% and resulted in a 3.7 times higher occurrence of panic disorder during the year following the attack (Wood et al., 2013).

Management of acute panic can be one of the most challenging aspects of PFA. Those who experience a panic attack have fears of dying, often by suffocation. Their attempts to get more air often lead to hyperventilation and actions of desperation that can endanger themselves or others. In most cases, the panic attack builds slowly as a crescendo of increasing arousal. PFA is most effective if it can be applied in the early stage of the attack, and a large part of its success is educating the person about what his or her body is doing and helping to normalize the response (i.e., it's not meant to harm).

Substance Use Disorders

People use a wide variety of both legal and illegal mood-altering substances in the wake of disaster, trauma, and general adversity. It's a form of self-medication designed to lessen the negative impact of the adversity. The DSM-5 identifies 10 classes of drugs (i.e., alcohol, caffeine, hallucinogens, inhalants, opioids, sedatives, hypnotics and anxiolytics, stimulants, tobacco, and other, often unknown substances), some of which are illegal, that individuals typically use despite problematic cognitive, behavioral, and psychological symptoms (American Psychiatric Association, 2013). Common features of substance use include impaired control over amounts and frequency, a desire to cut down on use, energy expended on acquiring the substance, cravings, impairment (social, occupational), risky use, continued use despite problems, increased tolerance, and withdrawal symptoms.

Excessive alcohol consumption is considered one of the leading preventable causes of death in the United States (Landen et al., 2014). The general 12-month prevalence rate of alcohol use in adults is estimated to be 8.5%, with rates noted to be higher for men (12.4%) than women (4.9%) (American Psychiatric Association, 2013). Moreover, alcohol-attributable mortality among American Indians and Alaska Natives was 10.3% in 2009 compared to 3.3% for whites (Landen et al., 2014). Data from a national longitudinal study of 2,316 participants revealed that alcohol use before 18 years of age was associated with significantly higher risk of future heavy alcohol use (five or more drinks per occasion), whereas abstinence from alcohol until age 18 years reduced risk of alcohol-related problems in adulthood (Liang & Chikritzhs, 2015). An 18-year trend study (1992, 2002, and 2010) of 9,207 16- and 17-year-old Norwegians showed an increase in alcohol measures from 1992 to 2002, followed by a decrease in the measures from 2002 to 2010. Over 18 years, alcohol use was negatively correlated with parental care, positively correlated with parents' binge drinking, and associated with symptoms of depression, tobacco use, and cannabis use (Pedersen & von Soest, 2015).

To generate the criteria to help assess an alcohol use disorder, the four-item **CAGE** questionnaire (Ewing, 1984) has been used for more than 30 years:

1. Have you ever felt the need to **C**ut down on your drinking?
2. Have you ever felt **A**nnoyed by criticism of your drinking?
3. Have you ever had **G**uilty feelings about your drinking?
4. Have you ever taken a morning **E**ye-opener (a drink to start the day)?

Two or more positive responses indicate alcohol-dependent behavior.

In a meta-analytic study of 31 population-based studies assessing substance use and misuse in the aftermath of terrorism, DiMaggio,

Galea, and Li (2009) reported that 7.3% of the population could be expected to report increased alcohol use in the first two years following a terrorist event (and that there is a 20% chance that the prevalence could be as high as 14%). The prevalence of cigarette smoking following a terrorist event could be expected to increase by 6.8% and mixed drug use (prescription medications and narcotics) might be expected to increase by 16.3%.

When PFA providers are working with emergency responders, it's also important to inquire not only about the use of alcohol but about energy drinks. Energy drinks are sympathomimetic stimulants (discussed in the next section) capable of inducing generalized, potentially excessive arousal. Sleep disturbance, anxiety, difficulty concentrating, tachycardia, and arrhythmias are possible consequences of overuse.

Unique Impact of the Covid-19 Pandemic

It is worth noting that the inevitable, if not imminent, outbreak of a viral pandemic was predicted a dozen years ago (Perrin et al., 2009). However, despite this warning, no one could have predicted the gravity and devastating impact of COVID-19, which will be addressed more in the following chapter. The physical and emotional impact has been unprecedented, as evidenced in part by how COVID-19 has adversely affected the prevalence rates of several of the syndromes just addressed.

For instance, according to a study of 5,470 respondents supported by the Centers for Disease Control and Prevention, Czeisler et al. (2020) reported that the prevalence of anxiety disorder symptoms in June 2020 increased more than three times the prevalence reported in the second quarter of 2019 (25.5% versus 8.1%) and the prevalence of depressive disorder approached four times that reported in the second quarter of 2019 (24.3% versus 6.5%). In the same study, the authors reported that symptoms of trauma-and-stressor-related disorder (which includes PTSD, acute stress disorder, and adjustment disorders) related to the pandemic had a rate of 26.3%, and 13.3% reported starting or increasing substance use as a coping mechanism for the stress of the pandemic. These immediate mental health implications clearly warrant concern and suggest that the full impact of COVID-19 on mental health might not be known for years. A putative reason for the impact COVID-19 has had on these prevalence rates, as well as on the psychophysiological stress syndromes described next, is that it has created a unique amalgam of "psychological toxicity" factors: severe impact (mortality, economic), prolonged duration (roughly 24 months), uncertainty regarding how to best mitigate the contagion effects, and a general lack of community resilience (politization, lack of community cohesion).

Psychophysiological Stress Reaction

The term *stress* was first used in the biological sciences in the 1930s by renowned endocrinologist Dr. Hans Selye (1974), who later in his career defined it as "the nonspecific response of the body to any demand made upon it" (p. 27). The most widely noted conceptual definition of stress, and one that is embedded in the vernacular, was formulated by physiologist Dr. Walter Cannon more than 100 years ago and referred to as the "fight or flight" response (Cannon, 1914). Cannon's concept is useful because it explains what the stress response was intended to do—to prepare you to fight or flee from a life-threatening event. If we consider a threatening, critical incident to be a toxin that affects the body and the mind, then a primary antidote to this toxin is to give people information to help them account for what is happening to them. Therefore, a working knowledge of the human nervous system and its physiological and psychological effects will enhance PFA providers' ability to help mitigate adverse reactions.

The human nervous system is divided into the central nervous system (brain and spinal cord) and the peripheral nervous system (that which lies outside the central nervous system). The peripheral nervous system is divided into the somatic nervous system, which is responsible for voluntary muscle movements, and the autonomic nervous system (ANS), which is involved in regulating the body's internal function and is associated primarily with the stress response. To prepare a person to fight or to flee, the body releases numerous and varied physiological mechanisms (see Everly & Lating, 2019, for a thorough description). There are three primary systems, or axes, that facilitate the expression of the human stress response.

The most rapid response comes from the neural axis and its accompanying pathways, which, in addition to the neuromuscular nervous system, contains the sympathetic nervous system (SNS) and the parasympathetic nervous system (PNS), both of which are part of the ANS. The SNS and PNS send neurochemical signals via neurotransmitters that affect your organs, muscles, and brain. The SNS and PNS work in concert, but in opposite directions, to maintain homeostasis within the body and help us survive. While the SNS is associated with the fight-or-flight response, the PNS is often referred to as the rest-and-digest response.

The SNS is responsible for common stress responses, such as dilating pupils to enhance vision, increasing heart rate to pump more blood to large muscles to provide more oxygen, diverting blood away from skin by constricting blood vessels (so you will bleed less if you are cut), and causing the liver to release glycogen, which is converted to glucose for energy (which, in turn, raises body temperature). This, for example, is why people often describe breaking out in a cold sweat when stressed (blood, which is warm, is not flowing to the periphery, so extremities, such as hands, are cold, and they are sweaty because of the rise in body temperature). In addition, the SNS limits activity of your digestive system during stress because digesting food at this time is not an efficient use of critical energy (as noted, your energy and physiological resources are focused on large muscles to help you fight or flee). The shutting down of the digestive system helps to explain phenomena such as "butterflies" in the stomach (which is the sensation of blood pooling out of the stomach) as well as the dry, cotton mouth one experiences under considerable stress (the production of saliva, which is the initial part of the digestive process, is appreciably reduced). When the threat subsides, the PNS slows the heart rate because the need to transport large amounts of oxygen is reduced. The PNS also activates and moderates your digestive system.

Moreover, excessive SNS activation, which occurs in the middle, more primitive functioning part of the brain that relies on basic reactions such as fight or flight, limits higher-order cognitive functioning that occurs in the front part of the brain. This results in a phenomenon known as *cortical inhibition* in which your ability to problem solve, let alone think clearly, is compromised. Unfortunately, the inability to think clearly during a stressful situation can further escalate heart rate, creating an unwanted, additive cycle.

Stress-induced heart rates around 115 to 120 beats per minute (bpm) may result in loss of fine-motor control, such as writing. However, at heart rates between 115 and 145 bpm, complex motor skills, such as shooting a gun or running into a fire with equipment, and cognitive functioning are at their peak (Grossman, 2008; McKay & McKay, 2013). Heart rates above 145 bpm are thought to lead to compromised cognitive ability, as well as decreased auditory and visual abilities, but gross-motor skills, such as running and lifting, remain optimal. Heart rates above 175 bpm can lead to disintegration of all skilled tasks, including physical and cognitive breakdowns (Grossman, 2008). These data are for stress-induced, not exercise-induced, heart rates, and there is considerable individual variability.

The second system, the neuroendocrine axis and its accompanying pathways, involves the adrenal glands, which sit above the kidneys. The central core of the adrenal glands, known as the adrenal medullae, releases the catecholamines epinephrine (adrenaline) and norepinephrine (noradrenaline) into the systemic blood circulation to functionally continue arousal of the SNS. This effect can produce increased heart rate, blood pressure, muscle tension, and cholesterol and triglyceride levels.

The third system, the endocrine axis and its accompanying pathways, requires greater intensity to activate and results in the most chronic and prolonged responses. Therefore, a PFA provider might encounter these reactions several days, weeks, or even months after the critical incident. For example, the outer layer of the adrenal glands, known as the adrenal cortices, releases the hormones cortisol (which increases blood-sugar levels, can cause weight gain, and increases cravings for high-calorie foods, suppresses immune system functioning, produces gastrointestinal problems, sexual dysfunction, skin problems, and cardiovascular disease) and aldosterone (which causes sodium and fluid retention and therefore raises blood pressure). Other long-term endocrine responses include alterations in thyroid hormones, leading to hyperthyroidism-like reactions (nervousness and irritability, heart palpitations, excessive sweating, and weight loss), hypothyroidism-like reactions (fatigue, weakness, hair loss, weight gain, muscle cramps, and intolerance to cold temperatures), or alterations in gonadotropic hormones (which could impair reproductive function).

In addition to these stress-induced physiological effects, numerous psychological reactions are possible. The psychological as well as the physiological reactions reviewed are most likely predicated on a quote credited to Selye: "It is not what happens to you that matters, but how you take it." Mark Twain once noted, "I am an old man and have known a great many troubles, but most of them never happened." Finally, it has been suggested that stress, like beauty, is in the eye of the beholder. What do these statements have in common? We believe that the preponderance of stress occurs because of how we view the people, places, and things around us (see Everly & Lating, 2004, 2019). Therefore, the interpretations and meanings one assigns to critical incidents are essential in determining happiness and the ability to cope with adversity. These concepts will be developed and expanded in later chapters of this book, but the basic tenet is that helping someone to recognize the early warning signs of excessive stress may better prepare the person to manage these reactions and avert dysfunction. The purpose of the RAPID PFA model is to provide these skills.

KEY POINT SUMMARY

1. The six psychological syndromes and reactions relevant to those providing PFA in the wake of adversity are (1) PTSD, (2) major depressive disorder (3) generalized anxiety disorder, (4) panic disorder, (5) substance use, and (6) psychophysiological stress

reactions. It is worth noting that the COVID-19 pandemic has had a unique impact on the prevalence rates of several of these syndromes.

2. Our intention is not to provide a diagnostic manual but, rather, to sensitize readers to the syndromes they may encounter in the field while providing a rationale for the need to offer some form of psychological intervention other than psychotherapy. Our review is neither diagnostic nor comprehensive. However, it prepares the reader to better understand chapter 4, which reviews the large-scale situational context for PFA most relevant to the public health challenge and the anticipation of mental health surge. Raphael (1986) estimated that *25% of the affected population could benefit from PFA.*

3. While some people might experience severe symptoms that require a formal response and even possibly referral to the next level of care, most people in the aftermath of a disaster are resilient (Bonanno et al., 2010).

4. Regardless of the actual presentation of signs and symptoms of distress in the wake of adversity, do these symptoms reach the magnitude of impairment or dysfunction? With that in mind, each survivor's presenting symptoms and level of impairment should be evaluated, not on whether they satisfy the threshold for a formal diagnosis but, rather, on an individual basis and considered with regard to how any or all of the presenting signs and symptoms affect the person, specifically regarding the degree of functional impairment and interference with necessary activities of current life.

5. Evidence of significant impairment that interferes with one's ability to perform necessary activities of current life (childcare, self-care, disaster recovery, employment, etc.) for a significant period usually warrants access to a higher level of care than PFA.

6. Reactions in the wake of extreme adversity can be psychological, behavioral, and psychophysiological syndromes. The PFA interventionist must be sensitive to evidence of impairment in each domain. The interventionist must also keep in mind that

impairment may be context specific. For example, someone may be functional at work but impaired regarding family domestic responsibilities or vice versa.

7. Most relevant for the process of PFA intervention planning is Dr. Hans Selye's notion: "It is not what happens to you that matters, but how you take it." The preponderance of stress in one's life occurs because of how one views the people, places, and things around him or her (see Everly & Lating, 2004, 2019). One cannot necessarily control what happens, but one can certainly influence one's own reaction to what happens. This provides the opportunity for the PFA interventionist to stabilize and mitigate acute distress.

References

American Psychiatric Association. (1954). *Psychological first aid in community disasters.* Washington, DC: American Psychiatric Association.

American Psychiatric Association. (2013). *Diagnostic and statistical manual of mental disorders* (5th ed.). Washington, DC: American Psychiatric Association.

Bennett, P., Williams, Y., Page, N., Hood, K., Woollard, M., & Vetter, N. (2005). Associations between organizational and incident factors and emotional distress in emergency ambulance personnel. *British Journal of Clinical Psychology, 44,* 215–226. http://dx.doi.org/10.1348/014466505x29639.

Bonanno, G. A. (2004). Loss, trauma, and human resilience: Have we underestimated the human capacity to thrive after extremely aversive events? *American Psychologist, 59,* 20–28. http://dx.doi.org/10.1037/0003-066X.59.1.20.

Bonanno, G. A., Brewin, C. R., Kaniasty, K., & La Greca, A. M. (2010). Weighing the costs of disaster: Consequences, risks, and resilience in individuals, families, and communities. *Psychological Science in the Public Interest, 11,* 1–49. http://dx.doi.org/10.1177/1529100610387086.

Bovasso, G., & Eaton, W. (1999). Types of panic attacks and their association with psychiatric disorder and physical illness. *Comprehensive Psychiatry, 40,* 469–477. http://dx.doi.org/10.1016/S0010-440x(99)90092-5.

Bryant, R., & Harvey, A. (1995). Posttraumatic stress reactions in volunteer firefighters: Predictors of distress. *Journal of Nervous and Mental Disease, 183,* 267–271. http://dx.doi.org/10.1097/00005053-199504000-00014.

Cannon, W. B. (1914). The emergency function of the adrenal medulla in pain and the major emotions. *American Journal of Physiology, 33*, 356–372.

Cramer, V., Torgersen, S., & Kringlen, E. (2005). Quality of life and anxiety disorders: A population study. *Journal of Nervous and Mental Disease, 193*, 196–202. http://dx.doi.org/10.1097/01.NMD.0000154836.22687.13.

Czeisler, M. É., Lane, R. I., Petrosky, E., Wiley, J. F., Christensen, A., Njai, R., . . . Rajaratnam, S. M. W. (2020). Mental health, substance use, and suicidal ideation during the COVID-19 pandemic—United States, June 24–30, 2020. *Morbidity and Mortality Weekly Report (MMWR), 69*, 1049–1057. http://dx.doi.org/10.15585/mmwr.mm6932a1.

DiMaggio, C., Galea, S., & Li, G. (2009). Substance use and misuse in the aftermath of terrorism: A Bayesian meta-analysis. *Addiction, 104*, 894–904. http://dx.doi.org/10.1111/j.1360-0443.2009.02526.x.

Everly, G. S., Jr. (2013). *Fostering human resilience: A primer on resilient leadership, psychological first aid, psychological body armor and critical incident stress management.* Ellicott City, MD: Chevron.

Everly, G. S., Jr., & Lating, J. M. (2004). *Personality-guided therapy of post-traumatic stress disorder.* Washington, DC: American Psychological Association.

Everly, G. S., Jr., & Lating, J. M. (2019). *A clinical guide to the treatment of the human stress response* (4th ed.). New York, NY: Springer Nature.

Ewing, J. A. (1984). Detecting alcoholism: The CAGE questionnaire. *JAMA, 252*, 1905–1907. https://doi.org/10.1001/jama.252.14.1905.

Fazel, M., Wheeler, J., & Danesh, J. (2005). Prevalence of serious mental disorder in 7000 refugees resettled in western countries: A systematic review. *The Lancet, 365*, 1309–1314. http://dx.doi.org/10.1016/S0140-6736(05)61027-6.

Fried, E. I., & Nesse, R. M. (2015). Depression is not a consistent syndrome: An investigation of unique symptom patterns in the STAR*D study. *Journal of Affective Disorders, 172*, 96–102. http://dx.doi.org/10.1016/j.jad.2014.10.010.

Ganzini, L., McFarland, B. H., & Cutler, D. (1990). Prevalence of mental disorders after catastrophic financial loss. *Journal of Nervous and Mental Disease, 178*, 680–685. http://dx.doi.org/10.1097/00005053-199011000-00002.

Goodwin, R. D., Olfson, M., Feder, A., Fuentes, M., Pilowsky, D. J., & Weissman, M. M. (2001). Panic and suicidal ideation in primary care. *Depression and Anxiety, 14*, 244–246. http://dx.doi.org/10.1002/da.1074.

Grossman, D. (with Christensen, L. W.). (2008). *On combat: The psychology and physiology of deadly conflict in war and in peace* (3rd ed.). Millstadt, IL: Warrior Science Publications.

Hartley, T. A., Burchfiel, C. M., Fekedulegn, D., Andrew, M. E., &Violanti, J. M. (2011). Health disparities in police officers: Comparisons to the U.S. general population. *International Journal of Emergency Mental Health, 13,* 211–220.

Hartley, T. A., Violanti, J. M., Sarkisian, K., Andrew, M. E., & Burchfiel, C. M. (2013). PTSD symptoms among police officers: Associations with frequency, recency, and types of traumatic events. *International Journal of Emergency Mental Health, 15,* 241–254.

Hines, L. A., Sundin, J., Rona, R. J., Wessely, S., & Fear, N. T. (2014). Posttraumatic stress disorder post Iraq and Afghanistan: Prevalence among military subgroups. *Canadian Journal of Psychiatry, 59,* 468–479.

Hinton, D. E., & Lewis-Fernández, R. (2011). The cross-cultural validity of posttraumatic stress disorder: Implications for DSM-5. *Depression and Anxiety, 28,* 783–801. http://dx.doi.org/10.1002/da.20753.

Jonsson, A., Segesten, K., & Mattsson, B. (2003). Post-traumatic stress among Swedish ambulance personnel. *Emergency Medical Journal, 20,* 79–84. http://dx.doi.org/10.1136/emj.20.1.79.

Kaplan, H. I., & Sadock, B. J. (1996). *Pocket handbook of primary care psychiatry.* Baltimore, MD: Williams & Wilkins.

Kessler, R. C., Berglund, P., Demler, O., Jin, R., Koretz, D., Merikangas, R., . . . Wang, P. S. (2003). The epidemiology of major depressive disorder: Results from the National Comorbidity Survey Replication (NCS-R). *JAMA, 289,* 3095–3105. http://dx.doi.org/10.1001/jama.289.23.3095.

Kessler, R. C., Chiu, W., Demler, O., & Walters, E. (2005). Prevalence, severity, and comorbidity of 12-month DSM-IV disorders in the National Comorbidity Survey Replication. *Archives of General Psychiatry, 62,* 617–627. http://dx.doi.org/10.1001/archpsyc.62.6.617.

Kessler, R. C., Sonnega, A., Bromet, E., Hughes, M., & Nelson, C. B. (1995). Posttraumatic stress disorder in the National Comorbidity Survey. *Archives of General Psychiatry, 64,* 1048–1060. http://dx.doi.org/10.1001 /archpsyc.1995.03950240066012.

Kinley, D. J., Cox, B. J., Clara, I., Goodwin, R. D., & Sareen, J. (2009). Panic attacks and their relation to psychological and physical functioning in Canadians: Results from a nationally representative sample. *Canadian Journal of Psychiatry, 54,* 113–122.

Kinley, D. J., Walker, J. R., Mackenzie, C. S., & Sareen, J. (2011). Panic attacks and panic disorder in a population-based sample of active Canadian military personnel. *Journal of Clinical Psychiatry, 72,* 66–74. http://dx.doi.org /10.4088/JCP.09m05587blu.

Klein, E., Linn, S., Colin, V., Lang, R., Pollcak, S., & Lenox, R. H. (2013). Anxiety disorders among patients in a general emergency service in Israel. *Hospital & Community Psychiatry, 46*, 488–492.

Kupchik, M., Strous, R. D., Erez, R., Gonen, N., Weizman, A., & Spivak, B. (2007). Demographic and clinical characteristics of motor vehicle accident victims in the community general health outpatient clinic: A comparison of PTSD and non-PTSD subjects. *Depression and Anxiety, 24*, 244–250. http://dx.doi.org/10.1002/da.20189.

Landen, M., Roeber, J., Naimi, T., Nielsen, L., & Sewell, M. (2014). Alcohol-attributable mortality among American Indians and Alaska Natives in the United States, 1999–2009. *American Journal of Public Health, 104*, S343–S349. http://dx.doi.org/10.2105/AJPH.2013.301648.

Lawson, K. J., Rodwell, J. L., & Noblet, A. J. (2012). Mental health of a police force: Estimating prevalence of work-related depression in Australia without a direct national measure. *Psychological Reports, 110*, 743–752. http://dx.doi.org/10.2466/01.02.13.17.PR0.110.3.743-752.

Lewis-Fernández, R., Hinton, D. E., Laria, A. J., Patterson, E. H., Hofmann, S. G., Craske, M. G., ... Liao, B. (2010). Culture and the anxiety disorders: Recommendations for DSM-V. *Depression and Anxiety, 27*, 212–229. http://dx.doi.org/10.1002/da.20647.

Liang, W., & Chikritzhs, T. (2015). Age at first use of alcohol predicts the risk of heavy alcohol use in early adulthood: A longitudinal study in the United States. *International Journal of Drug Policy, 26*, 131–134. http://dx.doi.org/10.1016/j.drugpo.2014.07.001.

Mancini, A. D., & Bonanno, G. A. (2006). Resilience in the face of potential trauma: Clinical practices and illustrations. *Journal of Clinical Psychology: In Session, 62*, 971–985. http://dx.doi.org/10.1002/jclp.20283.

Marcus, M., Yasamy, M. T., van Ommeren, M., Chisholm, D., & Saxena, S. (2012). *Depression: A global public health concern.* Geneva, Switzerland: WHO Department of Mental Health and Substance Abuse. http://www.who.int/mental_health/management/depression/who_paper_depression_wfmh_2012.pdf.

Martin, M., Marchand, A., & Boyer, R. (2009). Traumatic events in the workplace: Impact on psychopathology and healthcare use of police officers. *International Journal of Emergency Mental Health, 11*, 165–176.

McKay, B., & McKay, K. (2013, August 15). Managing stress arousal for optimal performance: A guide to the warrior color code. *Art of Manliness* (blog). http://www.artofmanliness.com/2013/08/15/managing-stress-arousal-for-optimal-performance-a-guide-to-the-warrior-color-code.

Meyer, E. C., Zimering, R., Daly, E., Knight, J., Kamholz, B. W., & Gulliver, S. B. (2012). Predictors of posttraumatic stress disorder and other physiological symptoms in trauma exposed firefighters. *Psychological Services, 9,* 1–15. http://dx.doi.org/10.1037/a0026414.

Neria, Y., Nandi, A., & Galea, S. (2008). Post-traumatic stress disorder following disasters: A systematic review. *Psychological Medicine, 38,* 467–480. http://dx.doi.org/10.1017/S0033291707001353.

Norris, F. H., Friedman, M. J., Watson, P. J., Byrne, C. M., Diaz, E., & Kaniasty, K. (2002). 60,000 disaster victims speak: Part I. An empirical review of the empirical literature, 1981–2001. *Psychiatry: Interpersonal and Biological Processes, 65,* 207–239. http://dx.doi.org/10.1521/psyc.65.3.207.20173.

Ogle, C., Rubin, D., Berntsen, D., & Siegler, I. (2013). The frequency and impact of exposure to potentially traumatic events over the life course. *Clinical Psychological Science: A Journal of the Association for Psychological Science, 1,* 426–434. http://dx.doi.org/10.1177/2167702613485076.

Pedersen, W., & von Soest, T. (2015). Adolescent alcohol use and binge drinking: An 18-year trend study of prevalence and correlates. *Alcohol and Alcoholism, 50,* 219–225. http://dx.doi.org/10.1093/alcalc/agu091.

Perrin, P., McCabe, O. L., Everly, G. S, Jr., & Links, J. (2009). Preparing for an influenza pandemic: Mental health considerations. *Prehospital and Disaster Medicine, 24,* 223–230. http://dx.doi.org/10.1017/s1049023x00006853.

Raphael, B. (1986). *When disaster strikes: How individuals and communities cope with catastrophe.* New York, NY: Basic Books.

Ruzek, J. I., Brymer, M. J., Jacobs, A. K., Layne, C. M., Vernberg, E. M., & Watson, P. J. (2007). Psychological first aid. *Journal of Mental Health Counseling, 29,* 14–49. http://dx.doi.org/10.17744/mehc.29.1.5racqxjueafabgwp.

Sareen, J., Cox, B. J., Afifi, T. O., De Graff, R., Asmundson, G. J. G., ten Have, M., & Stein, M. B. (2005). Anxiety disorders and risk for suicidal ideation and suicide attempts: A population-based longitudinal study of adults. *Archives of General Psychiatry, 62,* 1249–1257. http://dx.doi.org/10.1001/arch psyc.62.11.1249.

Selye, H. (1974). *Stress without distress.* Philadelphia, PA: J. B. Lippincott.

Tracy, M., Morgenstern, H., Zivin, K., Aiello, A., & Galea, S. (2014). Traumatic event exposure and depression severity over time: Results from a prospective cohort study in an urban area. *Social Psychiatry and Psychiatric Epidemiology, 49,* 1769–1782. http://dx.doi.org/10.1007/s00127-014-0884-2.

Tully, P. J., & Baune, B. T. (2014). Comorbid anxiety disorders alter the association between cardiovascular diseases and depression: The German national health interview and examination survey. *Social Psychiatry and*

Psychiatric Epidemiology, 49, 683–691. http://dx.doi.org/10.1007/s00127-013 -0784-x.

Weissman, M. M., Bland, R. C., Canino, G. J., Faravelli, C., Greenwald, S., Hwu, H-G., . . . Yeh, E-K. (1996). Cross-national epidemiology of major depression and bipolar disorder. *JAMA, 276,* 293–299. http://dx.doi.org /10.1001/jama.1996.03540040037030.

Wood, C. M., Salguero, J. M., Cano-Vindel, A., & Galea, S. (2013). Perievent panic attacks and panic disorder after mass trauma: A 12-month longitudinal study. *Journal of Traumatic Stress, 26,* 338–344. http://dx.doi.org/10.1002 /jts.21810.

World Health Organization. (2020, January 30). *Depression* [Fact sheet]. Retrieved from https://www.who.int/en/news-room/fact-sheets/detail /depression.

Zinzow, H. M., Resnick, H. S., McCauley, J. L., Amstadter, A. B., Ruggiero, K. J., & Kilpatrick, D. G. (2012). Prevalence and risk of psychiatric disorders as a function of variant rape histories: Results from a national survey of women. *Social Psychiatry and Psychiatric Epidemiology, 47,* 893–902. http://dx.doi.org/10.1007/s00127-011-0397-1.

FOUR | In the Wake of Disaster
The Large-Scale Context for PFA

IN CHAPTER 3, WE REVIEWED the six most common psychological and behavioral syndromes that occur in the wake of traumatic incidents and disasters. These descriptions were largely generic and context free. It is not an unreasonable leap to say that the nature of and context within which adverse events occur shape the responses to those events. Disasters are a special case. By definition, disasters are overwhelming. They overwhelm our resources and often even our expectations. They might even serve to violate deeply held core beliefs. Such adversity cannot help but shape the syndromes described in the previous chapter. They sometimes even challenge our belief in our own capacity to help those in need. In this chapter, we take a closer look at disasters, as they will likely be the most challenging context within which PFA will be practiced. Some familiarity with various types of disasters and aspects of their psychological impact will better prepare you to respond within this context.

Types of Disasters

Most research on psychological effects of disasters focuses on a specific event or disaster, with the type of disaster falling into one of three categories: (1) natural, (2) technological, and (3) mass violence or terrorism (Neria, Nandi, & Galea, 2008). Natural disasters typically occur due to unexpected weather and geological events. The degree of destruction natural disasters wreak depends on a variety of factors, including the intensity of the event, the population density where the events occur, and the degree of preparation available, including architectural strength and established warning systems. Natural disasters are often thought to occur randomly, though there are regions in the world more prone to certain types of natural disasters, such as hurricanes in the southeast of the United States and the Caribbean and earthquakes in Asia. There were reported to be 416 worldwide natural disasters in 2020 (Statista, 2021), and according to Munich Re (2021), a German reinsurance company that monitors worldwide natural disasters, the economic toll of these, not including COVID-19, totaled $210 billion (US dollars). Technological disasters are defined as events caused by human beings but without intent to harm. In contrast, human-made events are defined by the element of intent to harm. This third category has received more attention since the beginning of this century because of repeated terrorist events and their effects.

Although these categorizations might initially seem arbitrary, the natural or man-made origin of an event and the presence or absence of intent to harm may be important factors in understanding how individuals and communities respond and recover. A comprehensive review of data from 284 reports of disaster-related posttraumatic stress disorder (PTSD) symptoms published between 1980 and 2008 revealed that the prevalence of PTSD is generally lower after natural disasters compared with human-made and technological disasters (Neria, Nandi, & Galea, 2008). This chapter describes the emotional symptoms and purported psychopathology that occurs in the aftermath of many of these salient disasters. Although reasonably comprehensive, it is not intended to be a methodological critique of the research reviewed, and space limitations require selectivity of incidents covered and is not intended to minimize the literature or occurrence of other notable events.

Natural Disasters

Hurricane Andrew, a category-four storm that later turned into a category-five hurricane, occurred on August 24, 1992, in the southern Florida Peninsula and south-central Louisiana and directly or indirectly killed 66 people, cost in excess of $25 billion in damages, and is one of the most-studied natural disasters in US history. A study of 61 survivors who lived in areas most affected by Hurricane Andrew conducted 6 to 12 months after the event revealed that 51% met criteria for a disorder that began after the hurricane, including probable PTSD in 36% of the sample, major depressive disorder (MDD) in 30%, and other anxiety disorders in 20%. More than 50% of the study participants had significant symptoms that persisted beyond months, and the risk factor most strongly associated with a poor mental health outcome was having sustained severe damage to home and property (David et al., 1996). Another study of community members living in the damaged neighborhoods assessed between one and four months after the hurricane reported that damage to dwelling, perceived loss, threat to life, and injury were the four hurricane-related variables most predictive of posttraumatic symptoms (Ironson et al., 1997).

Earthquakes and tsunamis are widely studied natural disasters but mostly outside of the United States. In the last 20 years, the December 26, 2004, earthquake in Indonesia that set off the massive Indian Ocean tsunami, the 2008 7.9-magnitude Sichuan (also Wenchuan) earthquake in China, the January 2010 earthquake in Haiti, and the 2011 Fukushima earthquake and tsunami in Japan have garnered the bulk of empirical attention. Within three to four weeks after the 2004 tsunami caused by a 9.0-magnitude earthquake that traveled in excess of 300 miles (480 kilometers) per hour and ravaged regions of South Asia and East Africa, killing more than 225,000 people and leaving more than 1.7 million homeless (Telford, Cosgrave, & Houghton, 2006), 14% to 39% of children living in severely affected areas of Sri Lanka met criteria for PTSD (Neuner et al., 2006). In another study four months after the tsunami, 41% of adolescents and 19.6% of their mothers had symptoms consistent with PTSD (Wickrama & Kaspar, 2007). In a study of adults 20 to 21 months after the tsunami, 21% of the sample reported clinically significant PTSD, 16% reported depression, and 30% reported anxiety (Hollifield et al., 2008). Exposure (e.g., thinking one's life was in danger, injury to family members, or death of family) was associated with increased impairment and respondents reported relying on their own strength, family, and religious practices to cope with their symptoms.

Hurricane Katrina, which made landfall in Louisiana on August 29, 2005, was one of the most devastating natural disasters in US history, killing more than 1,800 people, destroying more than 200,000 homes, and costing more than $100 billion in property damage (CNN Editorial Research, 2021; Deryugina, Kawano, & Levitt, 2018; Rosenbaum, 2006). A representative sample of 1,043 people in areas affected by Hurricane Katrina revealed estimated prevalence rates of PTSD of 30% of those residing in the New Orleans metropolitan area and 12% for those residing in Alabama, other parts of Louisiana, and Mississippi (Galea et al., 2007). In a study of 815 affected residents conducted five to eight months after Hurricane Katrina, and followed up one year later, it was found that contrary to expectations that mental health would improve over time, the prevalence of PTSD increased in the total sample from 14.9% to 20.9%, serious mental illness increased from 10.9% to 14.0%, and suicidal ideation increased from 2.8% to 6.4% (Kessler et al., 2008). The authors note that unresolved stress related to the effects of Katrina accounted for the preponderance of the increases over time. The ability to help resolve acute stress is a primary goal of PFA.

In a unique study that assessed psychological symptoms as part of ongoing clinical care in 76 patients at an outpatient psychiatric clinic one month prior to Hurricane Katrina and in 80 patients one month after Katrina made landfall, it was found that depression scores increased significantly, but there were no differences in PTSD scores (possibly due to being assessed too soon after the event). Depressive symptoms were related to the amount of time spent watching television coverage of the looting that occurred and the amount of time being without electricity (McLeish & Del Ben, 2008). In a study conducted eight weeks after Hurricane Katrina, 26% of a sample of 912 New Orleans Police Department (NOPD) personnel who provided law enforcement and relief services to impacted communities after Katrina reported symptoms consistent with depression, and 19% reported symptoms consistent with PTSD. In this same study, depressive symptoms were associated with minimal family contact, uninhabitable homes, injury to a family member, and isolation from the NOPD, whereas PTSD symptoms were associated with recovery of bodies, crowd control, assault, and injury to one's family (West et al., 2008). From a PFA perspective, and consistent with other literature, lack of support and exposure to distressing events, including watching too much television related to the traumatic event (Propper et al., 2007), can have adverse effects.

In a study of 704 survivors one year after the 2008 Sichuan earthquake in China, also referred to as the Wenchuan earthquake, in which a 7.9-magnitude quake resulted in more than 87,000 deaths and 4.8 million homeless, it was found that 23.0% and 13.8% of the survivors had moderate and severe depression, respectively, and that depression severity was higher in severely damaged, compared to moderately damaged, areas (Xu, Mo, & Wu, 2013). Four months after the 2010, 7.0-magnitude earthquake in Haiti, in which approximately 300,000 people died and more than 2 million were left homeless (Haitian Conference, 2010), the first population-based survey of 1,323 survivors selected randomly from displaced and nondisplaced settings revealed that more than 90% had at least one relative or close friend killed and 93% reported seeing dead bodies. The prevalence of PTSD in this sample was 24.6%, and job loss and low social support following the earthquake were associated with increased risk. The prevalence of MDD for the sample was 28.3%, and during the earthquake, major damage to one's home was associated with higher MDD risk. Following the earthquake, mental illness of a family member increased risk (Cerdá et al., 2013). A disconcerting yet compounding psychosocial consequence in the aftermath of the Haitian earthquake, and one that has been noted previously in the literature (Clemens et al., 1999; Curtis, Miller, & Berry, 2000; Rashid, 2000), was the epidemic rise of sexual violence against women (Center for Human Rights and Global Justice, 2011), with estimates of sexual violence ranging between 50% and 72%

(Willman & Marcelin, 2010). In a focus group using a semistructured questionnaire with 16 women between ages 19 and 52 years who self-identified as victims of sexual violence in the Cité Soleil, Haiti, Rahill et al. (2015) reported endorsed criteria consistent with PTSD.

The Great East Japan Earthquake, which measured 9.0 on the Richter scale, struck the northeastern part of Japan on March 11, 2011, at around 2:36 p.m. About an hour after the earthquake, a massive tsunami with 30-foot waves ravaged Japan's coastline. The tsunami, along with additional earthquake aftershocks, caused explosions and cooling system failures at the Fukushima Daini and Fukushima Daiichi power plants, resulting in massive evacuations. The incident killed close to 16,000 people, destroyed more than 400,000 homes, resulted in the evacuation of close to 185,000 people, and cost more than $300 billion in damages (Sakuma et al., 2015). In a study of 241 evacuees from Hirono, Fukushima, 33.2% indicated probable symptoms of PTSD, and 19.1% and 14.5% demonstrated moderate and severe depressive symptoms, respectively (Kukihara et al., 2014). In a study assessing 610 local municipality workers (e.g., involved in restoration activities, managing evacuation centers and temporary morgues, and disaster debris disposal), 421 hospital medical workers, and 327 firefighters 14 months after the earthquake, it was found that 6.6%, 6.6%, and 1.6%, respectively, met criteria for probable PTSD; 15.9%, 14.3%, and 3.8%, respectively, met criteria for probable depression; and 14.9%, 14.5%, and 2.6%, respectively, met criteria for general psychological distress (Sakuma et al., 2015). Lack of communication was associated with increased risk of PTSD and depression in municipality and medical workers; lack of rest was correlated with increased risk of PTSD and depression in the municipality and medical workers; and for the municipality workers, increased risk for PTSD and depression was associated with disaster-related work. To place some of these data in context, the 12-month prevalence rate of PTSD in the general population of Japan is 0.4%, and the 12-month prevalence rate of major depression in the general population of Japan is 3% (Kawakami et al., 2005).

On October 29, 2012, Hurricane Sandy made landfall in the most densely populated region in the United States and affected an estimated 60 million people, resulting in more than 200,000 damaged or destroyed homes, costing an estimated $50 billion (Neria & Shultz, 2012; Walsh & Schwartz, 2012). In a study of 200 adults six months after the storm who lived in 18 beach communities in Monmouth County, New Jersey, it was found that 14.5% screened positive for PTSD and 6.0% met criteria for major depression. The variables most strongly associated with PTSD were high hurricane exposure and having high environmental health concerns (e.g., exposure to sewage, pollution, chemicals, or debris), whereas depression was most strongly associated with having physical limitations (Boscarino et al., 2013).

Since the publication of the first edition of this book, the outbreak of the novel severe acute respiratory syndrome coronavirus 2 (SARS-CoV-2) (Wiersinga & Prescott, 2020), better known now as COVID-19, rapidly morphed into a pandemic (*pan* derived from the Greek for "all" and *demos* for "people") after experts believe it first began infecting humans in late 2019 in Wuhan, a city in the Hubei Province of China (Velavan & Meyer, 2020). The global impact of COVID-19 has been profound. The Johns Hopkins University & Medicine (2021) Coronavirus Resource Center has noted that the worldwide prevalence of infection has exceeded 366 million cases, and the worldwide COVID-19-related death toll has exceeded 5.6 million people, with over 878,000 of those deaths occurring in the United States. Harvard economists have estimated that the cumulate economic toll of COVID-19 in the United States alone, including loss of life, loss of output, reduced quality of life, and mental health conditions, will exceed a staggering $16 trillion (Cutler & Summers, 2020). An additional notable, if not alarming, aspect of these daunting US numbers is the disproportionately higher rates of infection, hospitalization, and death of Black, Hispanic, and Asian people compared to White people (Lopez, Hart, & Katz, 2021).

The unprecedented public health measures deemed necessary to mitigate the spread of this highly infectious virus have resulted in emotional symptoms in survivors, family members, and the extended community, such as isolation and loneliness, physical and emotional fatigue, and feeling overwhelmed by media inundation, job loss, and financial concerns (Holmes et al., 2020; Lai et al., 2020). In addition, many of the formal mental health conditions noted in the previous chapter, such as anxiety, depression, PTSD, panic, and suicide, have been noted to occur (Lei et al., 2020; Moghanibashi-Mansourieh, 2020; Pappa et al., 2020). While no one has been spared from the possible effects of COVID-19, there has been particular concern for those consistently exposed to the virus, most notably health care workers. In what is considered the first study assessing the psychological symptoms of Chinese frontline health care workers (i.e., doctors, nurses, and support staff) in Wuhan during the COVID-19 pandemic, Du et al. (2020) reported that 12.7% had elevated depressive scores, 20.1% had anxiety symptoms, and 59% had moderate to severe levels of perceived stress. A more recent study on a sample of 304 health care workers in Shanghai found that 27.6% met criteria for probable PTSD (Yin et al., 2021). In a study assessing the impact of COVID-19 on 898 US young adults with ages ranging from 18 to 30 years, Liu et al. (2020) reported that 43.3% of the sample had symptoms consistent with depression, 45.4% had high anxiety scores, and 31.8% had symptoms consistent with probable PTSD. Of note, high levels of loneliness, worrying about COVID-19, and low tolerance for distress were associated with the observed levels of depression, anxiety, and PTSD symptoms. In a meta-analysis with a total sample size of 189,159 that focused on the mental health consequences of COVID-19, Cénat et al. (2021) reported that the prevalence of depression was 15.97%, the prevalence of anxiety was 15.15%, and the prevalence of PTSD was 21.94%.

Technological Disasters

Technological disasters are less widely studied but still have a major impact on the psychological health of the affected community. The 1979 Three Mile Island (TMI) nuclear power plant accident that occurred in Pennsylvania is one of the first examples of a technological disaster investigated for its lasting mental health effects. It was also my (GSE's) first disaster deployment. Much of the research on this disaster has focused on the acute and chronic physical effects of radiation and radioactive material exposure. Although continuing surveillance has not found consistent evidence of an increase in mortality or severe morbidity resulting from the radiation exposure (Talbott et al., 2003), several studies have found increases in various mental health problems in both the short and long term. A study a few months after the accident of 403 persons living within 5 miles of TMI and 1,506 people living within 55 miles of the area revealed elevated levels of general psychological symptoms among adults who lived close to the site, as compared with adults living farther away (Cleary & Houts, 1984). A study of 110 mothers with infants found that rates of general anxiety disorder and MDD were 15% to 18% among those living near the plant compared to 7% to 11% among mothers living farther away (Dew & Bromet, 1993).

Consistent with these findings were those of Davidson and Baum (1986), who found that five years after the accident residents living within 5 miles of TMI had persistent symptoms of PTSD and higher baseline values of heart rate and blood pressure compared to residents living 80 miles away. In October 1985, six years following the accident, the TMI nuclear-generating facility was restarted. Prince-Embury and Rooney (1988) assessed 108 residents in the vicinity of TMI after this restart to address its impact, and their results revealed that "those worried about developing cancer who psychologically distanced themselves from the fact of restart, who had lost trust in experts, and who accepted restart because they could not change it reported significantly more symptoms" (p. 789). These results depict the adverse and enduring impact that limited information, along with perceived lack of safety, trust, and control, can have on people. Norris et al. (2002), in their review of the disaster literature, concluded that the population affected by the TMI disaster was chronically stressed by the uncertainty associated with exposure effects and that this stress put them at increased risk for psychopathological symptoms.

The April 26, 1986, Chernobyl (Russian spelling), or Chornobyl (Ukrainian spelling), Nuclear Power Plant explosion in Ukraine (formerly part of the Soviet Union), in which an explosion of a reactor resulted in a fire that lasted for 10 days and emitted huge amounts of radioactive materials, created arguably the worst nuclear disaster the world has ever seen, accompanied by daunting public health problems (Loganovsky et al., 2008). In the years since the catastrophe, there have been numerous studies assessing its psychological impact. In a study comparing 1,617 participants who live in Gomel (close to Chernobyl) with 1,427 participants who live in Tver (500 miles from the disaster) six years after the event, Havenaar et al. (1997) reported that rates of *DSM-III-R* (American Psychiatric Association, 1987) mood disorders were 16.5% in Gomel versus 12.8% in Tver, whereas *DSM-III-R* anxiety disorders were 18.5% in Tver versus 12.6% in Gomel. However, PTSD prevalence was higher in Gomel (2.4%) than in Tver (0.4%). None of these differences was statistically significant. When 295 male cleanup workers—who were sent to Chernobyl for the initial cleanup, initially assessed, and then interviewed again 18 years after the accident—were compared with 397 matched controls who were initially assessed and then interviewed 16 years after the accident, it was found that after the accident, more cleanup workers than controls experienced depression (18.0% vs. 13.1%). When both groups were interviewed and assessed years later, rates of depression (14.9% vs. 7.1%), PTSD (4.1% vs. 1.0%), other anxiety disorders (5.1% vs. 3.0%), and headaches (69.2% vs. 12.4%) were significantly higher for the cleanup workers compared to controls (Loganovsky et al., 2008). In a sample of 321 immigrants to the United States after the Chernobyl incident, it was shown that geographic proximity to the event resulted in poor self-perceived health, depression, anxiety, and posttraumatic stress (Foster & Goldstein, 2007). In a 25-year retrospective of the Chernobyl disaster, Bromet, Havenaar, and Guey (2011) noted that mental health effects were the most prominent public health consequence resulting from the incident.

The 1989 *Exxon Valdez* oil spill disaster off the coast of Alaska occurred when the tanker ran aground and spilled at least 11 million gallons of crude oil, resulting in extensive environmental and ecological damage (Gill, Picou, & Ritchie, 2011) and adversely affecting the surrounding community, even though it did not place survivors in immediate physical danger or risks of personal danger. In a study of 599 participants conducted one year after the spill, rates of probable PTSD of 9.4% and rates of generalized anxiety of 20.2% were reported. In the same study, those with the greatest exposure (property damage, direct contact with the oil spill, etc.) were 3.6 times more likely to have generalized anxiety disorder (GAD), 2.9 times more likely to have PTSD, and 1.8 times more likely to have depression when compared with those not exposed (Palinkas et al., 1993).

On April 20, 2010, the *Deepwater Horizon*, an oil rig that was drilling an exploratory well 18,360 feet below sea level and roughly 41 miles off the Louisiana coast, ignited and exploded, engulfing the platform, killing 11 of the 126 crew members, and injuring 17 others. The incident was compounded over the course of the next 87 days, when approximately 185 million to 205 million gallons of crude oil were released before the well was capped on July 15 and permanently sealed on September 19, making it the biggest oil spill in US history (Gill, Picou, & Ritchie, 2011; Robertson & Krauss, 2010; Shenesey & Langhinrichsen-Rohling, 2015). In assessing the immediate psychological impact of the *Deepwater Horizon* oil spill in a sample of 588 Gulf Coast residents, 28% indicated significant levels of PTSD symptoms (Mong, Noguchi, & Ladner, 2012). In a study of 1,119 adult clients receiving services in various mental health agencies on the Gulf Coast of Mississippi, 36.6% noted a worsening of their financial situation, 23.6% reported worsening social relationships, 24.3% noted worsened physical health, and 39.1% reported symptoms consistent with probable PTSD (with those experiencing worsened financial situations and social relationships reporting more PTSD symptoms) (Drescher, Schulenberg, & Smith, 2014). In a study comparing psychological distress between 23 residents of fishing communities who were directly impacted by the spill (living or working in a community where spilled oil reached the shoreline) with 71 residents indirectly impacted, as well as comparing 47 residents who reported income stability following the spill with 47 residents who reported spill-related income loss, socioeconomic factors had the greatest impact. For example, depression scores were elevated in both groups (30% income stable, 62% income loss), but they were significantly higher in the income loss group. Consistent with this finding, 24% of people in the income stable group reported tension or anxiety compared to 65% of those in the income loss group (Grattan et al., 2011).

The 2011 earthquake and resulting tsunami in Japan also led to a Level 7 meltdown on the International Nuclear Event Scale at the Fukushima Daiichi Nuclear Power Plants; the nearby Fukushima Daini plant experienced substantial damage but remained operative. In an assessment of workers from the Daiichi (N = 885) and Daini (N = 610) plants two to three months after the disaster, it was found that the Daiichi workers compared to the Daini workers had higher rates of psychological distress (47% vs. 37%) and higher rates of posttraumatic stress response (30.0% vs. 19.0%). Shigemura et al. (2012) noted that discrimination or slurs (the electric company was criticized for their disaster response and workers received derogatory slurs) were associated with both high psychological distress and high posttraumatic stress response in the workers.

A unique twist to the 2011 nuclear disaster in Japan is that for many of the elderly it was thought to rouse memories and anxiety reactions of the World War II atomic bomb attacks on Hiroshima and Nagasaki (McCartney, 2011). Because parental distress is thought to be transferred to offspring through maladaptive communication and behaviors (Wiseman, Metzl, & Barber, 2006; Yehuda et al., 2008), Palgi et al. (2012) tested this possibility in grandchildren of A-bomb survivors and found that those whose grandparents had lived in the area of Hiroshima or Nagasaki and were exposed to the attacks exhibited a higher risk of probable PTSD (54.5%), more ruminations about the World War II attacks, and increased worries about future disasters compared to a control group whose grandparents were not exposed to the World War II attacks. In addition, perceived stigma and discrimination against those with radiation exposure has occurred in Japan since the Hiroshima and Nagasaki attacks (Tone & Stone, 2014), and Ben-Ezra et al. (2015) tested the association between radiation stigma and PTSD symptoms across geographic regions of Japan with a history of radiation exposure. In their study assessing participants from Hiroshima and Nagasaki (N = 253), Tokyo (N = 251), and Fukushima (N = 246), probable PTSD prevalence was 10.6% in Fukushima, compared to 2.4% in Tokyo and Hiroshima and Nagasaki, and the Fukushima group endorsed more radiation stigma perception compared to the other groups.

Human-Made Disasters

Disasters resulting from human actions undertaken with the intent to harm are usually referred to as mass violence or terrorism. Mass violence is often associated with isolated or premeditated shooting sprees, whereas terrorism is typically defined as a means of inducing fear and intimidation to generate negative psychological effects in the targeted population (Martino, 2002). As noted by Friedland and Merari (1985), "Terrorism bears primarily on the individual's perceptions, on the 'public mind'; in other words, it is a form of psychological warfare" (p. 592). In addition to the immediate impact of a specific event, terrorism is also characterized by the persistent threat of more violence, which may lead to different emotional outcomes in the long-term from other types of disasters. For example, bioterrorism is associated with our most fundamental fears of disease and death. Bioterrorist events, because of their possible invisible nature, extreme lethality, long incubation time, and lack of defined perimeter, expose our societal vulnerability. An intentional biochemical or chemical terrorist attack using agents such as inhalation anthrax, botulism, plague, smallpox, tularemia, sarin, or a combination of these or other agents will clearly have profound medical effects. Yet the psychological impact in the aftermath of a bioterrorist attack may be equally daunting. Estimates suggest that, for every one physical illness produced by a biological or chemical agent, between 50 and 100 individuals will experience psychological distress at a level that impairs their daily functioning (DeMartino, 2002).

Consider, for example, the outcome of the sarin gas attacks by the Aum Shinrikyo cult in a crowded Tokyo subway in March 1995. Cult members placed sealed plastic bags of diluted sarin onto the subway trains and then pierced the bags with sharpened umbrella tips before leaving the train (Bowler, Murai, & True, 2001). In addition to the physical injuries and symptoms reported from the attacks, which included cardiac problems, neuropathy, nausea, eye irritation, coughing, and headaches, there were considerable symptoms of psychological distress, especially because the substance (i.e., sarin) was not identified for three hours. Within weeks of the attacks, 60% of surveyed victims had symptoms consistent with PTSD (nightmares, flashbacks, intrusion, and avoidance) (Asukai, 1999), and four years after the attacks, 57% of victims who responded to a survey continued to have symptoms of depression, flashbacks, nightmares, and panic when boarding trains (Watts, 1999). Watts reported that lack of knowledge about the long-term effects of sarin gas added to the public's already heightened sense of distress. Ohbu et al. (1997) studied 641 patients on the day of the disaster and reported that 531 patients (83%) were classified as *mild*, meaning they were treated in the outpatient department and released after six hours of observation. According to Ursano et al. (2003), the preponderance of the 5,500 patients who sought medical care had no sign of exposure, and "many misattributed the signs and symptoms of anxiety and autonomic arousal to intoxication by sarin" (p. 142).

Within a month of the sarin gas attacks in Tokyo, the truck-bomb explosion of the Alfred P. Murrah Federal Building in Oklahoma City on April 19, 1995, resulted in the deaths of 168 people, including 19 children, and nearly 700 more injured. More than 800 buildings in the area were destroyed or damaged, with an estimated property damage of $625 million (North et al., 1999). Until September 11, 2001, the Oklahoma City bombing had been the worst terrorist attack to take place in the United States. Six months after the bombing, a study of 182 adult survivors found that 34.3% met criteria for PTSD and 45% met criteria for a postdisaster psychiatric disorder. In this study, women had higher rates of PTSD, major depression, and GAD compared to men and were more likely to meet criteria for some postdisaster diagnosis. The researchers also found that 63% of those individuals with any postdisaster diagnosis had a history of at least one lifetime psychiatric diagnosis (North et al., 1999).

A study of 494 survivors between 18 and 36 months after the bombing found that 28% suffered from anxiety and 26% met diagnostic criteria for depression, with higher rates of these disorders among those who were hospitalized after the event (Shariat et al., 1999). A study of posttraumatic symptoms six months after the bombing identified a variety of factors that increased an individual's risk for continuing symptoms. These factors include sustaining injuries during the bombing, feeling nervous or afraid at the time of the bombing, and reporting symptoms of arousal at the time of the event. Feelings of nervousness or fear were the most powerful predictors, followed by the fear of dying and being upset by others' reactions to the event (Tucker et al., 1997). Nearly three years after the incident, male primary victims of the direct bomb blast and male rescue workers (i.e., firefighters) who responded to the bombing were assessed with the same diagnostic interview. The results revealed higher rates of PTSD in male primary victims (23%) compared to male rescue workers (13%) and higher rates of postdisaster panic disorder in male primary victims (5%) compared to male rescue workers (1%); however, the rate of alcohol use disorder was higher in the rescue workers (25%) than in the primary victims (10%). PTSD affected individuals who spent more time at the bombing site, and more than half of the firefighters had a preexisting disorder, with alcohol abuse/dependency occurring in 47% of these cases (North et al., 2002).

The attacks of September 11, 2001—in which two hijacked airliners were flown into the New York City World Trade Center (WTC) towers, a third plane hit the Pentagon outside of Washington, DC, and a fourth plane crashed in a field in Pennsylvania—resulted in more than 3,000 deaths, including at least 400 police officers and firefighters (History Channel, 2018). In the 10 years following these terrorist attacks, there were more than 150 studies assessing its mental health effects (Perlman et al., 2011). Here we review a sampling of those findings.

In a random telephone sample of 1,008 adults who lived south of 110th Street in Manhattan (which is approximately eight miles north of the WTC), interviewed between five and nine weeks after the attacks, Galea et al. (2002) found that 7.5% of the participants reported symptoms of PTSD and 9.7% reported symptoms of depression, whereas 20.0% of the sample living south of Canal Street (nearer the WTC) reported PTSD symptoms. In another study, Schlenger et al. (2002), in a web-based survey of 2,273 adults, reported PTSD prevalence rates of 11.2% in New York City, 2.7% in Washington, DC, 3.6% in other major metropolitan areas, and 4.0% for the rest of the country.

Several explanations have been offered for the lower rates occurring in Washington, DC. One observation is that the general population interpreted the attack on the Pentagon as aimed at a military target and therefore less personally relevant than the civilian target of the WTC, where a common response might have been, "This could have happened to me."

Using data from the World Trade Center Health Registry (WTCHR), a longitudinal cohort of close to 29,000 highly exposed individuals to the WTC attack (residents near the WTC, persons who were in Lower Manhattan during the attacks, schoolchildren and staff, and rescue/recovery workers), investigators reported overall prevalence rates of PTSD two to three years after the attacks to be 12.4% among rescue/recovery workers, ranging from 6.2% for police to 12.2% for firefighters to 11.6% for emergency medical services personnel to as high as 21.2% for unaffiliated volunteers (including clergy and individuals in occupations unrelated to rescue and recovery work). Significant risk factors for PTSD in this sample included an earlier start date for work after the attacks, amount of time spent working at the WTC site, and performing tasks not typical of their occupation (e.g., the strongest risk factor for probable PTSD in the unaffiliated workers was firefighting) (Perrin et al., 2007). In a sample of more than 10,000 WTC workers assessed over a five-year period, it was found that 11.1% of the sample met criteria for probable PTSD, 8.8% met criteria for depression, 5.0% met criteria for panic disorder, and 17% were classified as having a probable alcohol problem. In addition, among those with probable PTSD, 12.7% also met criteria for a panic disorder or depression. It was also notable that unlike the Kessler et al. (2008) study from Hurricane Katrina, the point prevalence of PTSD, as expected, declined from 13.5% to 9.7% over the five years of assessment (Stellman et al., 2008).

In a study of 1,453 participants two years after the attacks, assessing whether negative beliefs related to terrorism (e.g., pessimism about world peace, feeling less safe than before 9/11) were related to distress (not using DSM diagnoses) and problematic drinking patterns, Richman et al. (2009) found that higher negative belief scores were significantly related to increased symptoms of depression, hostility, anxiety, somatization, and PTSD, along with an increase in binge drinking and escapist motives (e.g., to feel less tense, to cheer up, to forget worries). In another study using the WTCHR database to assess the frequency of binge drinking (consuming five or more drinks on five or more occasions in the past 30 days) five to six years after exposure to 9/11, the results revealed that binge drinking was significantly higher among those with PTSD (14.8%) compared to those without PTSD (6.3%). Moreover, those with *very high* and *high* WTC exposure (a summary measure of 12 events, such as being in the North or South WTC tower or another collapsed building at the time of the attack, fear of being killed, having a relative, friend, or coworker killed) had a higher prevalence of frequent binge drinking (13.7% and 9.8%, respectively) compared with those with medium or low exposure (7.5% and 4.4%, respectively) (Welch et al., 2014).

In a prospective cohort study of more than 43,000 adults without a diagnosis of PTSD prior to September 11, 2001, and assessed two to three years and then five to six years after their exposure to the September 11 WTC terrorist attack, rates of probable PTSD went from 14.3% two to three years after the attacks to 19.1% five to six years after the attack. According to Landrigan et al. (2004), PTSD symptoms were related to intense dust cloud exposure, which was considered to be highly alkaline with particulate matter considered capable of causing respiratory irritation and damage; witnessing horrific events; sustaining an injury; and losing a loved one, coworker, or acquaintance as a result of the attack. PTSD symptoms were also related to job loss and low social support after the attack. In addition, co-occurrence of postevent asthma and symptoms of PTSD occurred in 36% of the sample (Brackbill et al., 2009). In a study assessing the 10-year course of PTSD and depression among disaster workers using data from the 29,000 enrollees in the WTCHR project (Caramanica et al., 2014), the results revealed that 15.2% reported symptoms indicative of PTSD, 14.9% reported symptoms of depression, and 10.1% reported both. Comorbid PTSD and depression were associated with high 9/11 exposures, low social integration, health-related unemployment, and experiencing one or more traumatic life events since 9/11.

Six years after the attacks of September 11, on April 16, 2007, 49 students and faculty at Virginia Polytechnic Institute and State University (Virginia Tech) were shot and 32 were killed in two episodes that occurred over a span of four hours, resulting in the deadliest school-shooting incident in US history. In the first systematic web-based survey of 4,639 students conducted three to four months after the shooting, 15.4% of respondents experienced probable PTSD, with women having a higher prevalence (23.2%) than men (9.9%). Moreover, inability to confirm safety of friends or the death of a friend or a close friend explained most of the high PTSD symptoms (Hughes et al., 2011).

On April 15, 2013, during the 117th Boston Marathon, two bombs exploded near the finish line, killing three spectators and wounding more than 280 other people (Gates et al., 2014). An intense four-day manhunt resulted in the killing of one suspect and the apprehension of another. In published data that address the emotional reaction to the incident, researchers assessed the response of 71 veterans (57.7% from the Vietnam War) who were part of an ongoing longitudinal study of PTSD at the VA Boston Healthcare System. Although average levels of PTSD symptom severity were not significantly different for the entire sample when assessed prebombing to postbombing, for the 42.3% who reported being personally affected by the experience, they showed increased symptoms of intrusive memories and nightmares and avoidance of stimuli associated with reported previous traumas (Miller et al., 2013).

From 2009 to July 2021, there have been an estimated 255 mass shootings (using the definition of a mass shooting as an incident in which four or more people are killed, excluding the shooter) in America, killing a cumulative 1,449 people and wounding 961 others (Everytown for Gun Safety Support Fund, 2021). Several of these have garnered national and international attention (and differing responses, including the use of PFA):

- The July 20, 2012, movie theater shooting in Aurora, Colorado, occurred when a 24-year-old gunman using semiautomatic weapons shot randomly into a crowded midnight showing of *The Dark Knight Rises*, killing 12 people and injuring 70 others.

- On December 14, 2012, in Newtown, Connecticut, a 20-year-old man shot and killed his 52-year-old mother as she slept in her bed and then, armed with several semiautomatic weapons, forced his way into the Sandy Hook Elementary School, where he killed 20 children, six adult staff members, and himself.

- On June 17, 2015, a 21-year-old gunman, with reported white supremacist beliefs, killed nine African Americans who were part of a Bible study group at Emanuel African Methodist Episcopal Church in Charleston, South Carolina.

- On June 12, 2016, a 29-year-old gunman opened fire at the Pulse nightclub in Orlando, Florida, killing 49 people and wounding 53 more.

- On October 1, 2017, a 64-year-old man opened fire upon the crowd attending a music festival in Las Vegas, Nevada. In a span of about 10 minutes, he fired more than 1,000 rounds of ammunition killing 58 people and injuring 869.

- On February 14, 2018, a 19-year-old gunman opened fire at Marjory Stoneman Douglas High School in Parkland, Florida, killing 17 people and injuring 17 more.

- On October 27, 2018, a 46-year-old gunman, who reportedly had posted anti-Semitic comments, killed 11 people and wounded six others at the Tree of Life synagogue in Pittsburgh, Pennsylvania.

- On August 3, 2019, a 21-year-old gunman, purportedly targeting Latinxs, opened fire at a Walmart in El Paso, Texas, killing 23 people and injuring at least 26 others. This incident was considered predicated on one of the most notable mass shootings outside of America that occurred on March 15, 2019, when a 28-year-old gunman attacked worshippers at two separate mosques, killing 51 and injuring 40 more in Christchurch, New Zealand.

The emotional impact in the aftermath of these and so many other mass-killing events is profound and has raised concerns about mental illness, access to firearms, hate crimes, employment screenings, and mental health policy (Leander, 2020; Rosenberg, 2014). The tragic repercussions of these shootings also indicate the imperative need for PFA interventions for primary, secondary, and tertiary victims.

War-Related Syndromes: A Special Case of Human-Made Disaster

The diagnosis of PTSD, which was officially codified in the *DSM-III* in 1980 by the American Psychiatric Association, was prompted by the experiences of returning Vietnam War veterans. The explicit diagnostic criteria of *DSM-III* enabled large-scale epidemiologic studies to occur that assessed PTSD prevalence rates in deployed and nondeployed veterans. From 1980 to 2009, a review of medical and psychological databases (e.g., Medline, PsychLit, Cochrane Library, National Library of Medicine) revealed that there have been more than 1,700 citations that meet the criteria by war era (e.g., Vietnam War, Persian Gulf War, Operation Iraqi Freedom [OIF], and Operation Enduring Freedom [OEF]), military status, deployment status, and study type that have assessed the prevalence of PTSD (Magruder & Yeager, 2009). In a systematic evaluative review of these possible citations, using stringent inclusion and exclusion criteria, Magruder and Yeager (2009) meta-analyzed 18 studies from these war eras. Their results revealed that the estimated prevalence of PTSD ranged from 4.7% to 19.9% among deployed OIF/OEF samples compared to 3.2% to 9.4% among the nondeployed comparison group, that PTSD ranged from 1.9% to 24.0% among deployed Persian Gulf War samples compared to 0.7% to 15.0% among the nondeployed comparison group, and that PTSD ranged from 8.5% to 19.3% among deployed Vietnam War samples compared to 1.1% to 12.9% among the nondeployed comparison group. In addition, these aggregate data indicate a 1.5 to 3.5 times increased risk for PTSD associated with deployment, regardless of the war era.

The focus for more than a decade has been on those returning from the wars in Iraq and Afghanistan. In Iraq alone, 4,418 US military personnel died and 31,994 were wounded in action (US Department of Defense, n.d.), along with 4,804 coalition military personnel (iCasualties, n.d.). From an economic perspective, the total US federal price tag for the post-9/11 wars in Iraq, Afghanistan, and Pakistan through fiscal year 2020 was estimated to be more than $6.4 trillion (Watson Institute International & Public Affairs, 2020). In these most recent wars, data suggest that risk for PTSD after deployment increased when military personnel witnessed killing or were responsible for killing; experienced threat of death, serious injury, or witnessed injury or death; or experienced diminished mental and physical health prior to combat (LeardMann et al., 2009; Maguen et al., 2010; Phillips et al., 2010). In a study of health problems among service members returning from OEF in Afghanistan ($N = 16,318$), OIF ($N = 222,620$), and other locations ($N = 64,967$), Hoge, Auchterlonie, and Milliken (2006) reported that 19.1% of soldiers who returned from OIF met risk criteria for a mental health concern, compared with 11.3% after Afghanistan, and 8.5% after other deployments. They also noted that two-thirds of service members who accessed mental health care did so within two months of returning home. However, in an earlier study, Hoge et al. (2004) reported that more than 60% of OIF veterans who screened positive for PTSD, generalized anxiety, or depression did not seek treatment.

There has also been a focus on mild traumatic brain injury (TBI) in military personnel returning from the recent wars. Mild TBI, defined in a study by Hoge et al. (2008, p. 453) as "an injury with loss of consciousness or altered mental status (e.g., dazed or confused)," was assessed in a sample of 2,525 Iraqi soldiers, and results showed that in the 124 soldiers reporting a loss of consciousness, 43.9% met criteria for PTSD, compared to 27.3% of the 260 who reported an injury with altered mental status, 16.2% of the 435 who reported some other injury, and 9.1% for the 1,706 who reported no injury. In a more recent study of 760 soldiers assessed before and after deployment to Iraq, of the 9% who acknowledged TBI, 17.6% screened positive for PTSD and 31.3% screened positive for depression (Vasterling et al., 2012).

There has been growing concern about suicide and suicidal ideation among military personnel. For instance, in a sample of 157 military personnel and four civilian contractors being evaluated and treated in Iraq for suspected head injury, the likelihood of previous suicidal ideation increased significantly with the number of TBIs, from none occurring in patients with no TBIs, to 6.9% with a single TBI, to 21.7% with those with multiple TBIs (Bryan & Clemans, 2013). In addition, data suggest that, in a study of 1,665 National Guard troops studied postdeployment, those who reported the most readjustment stressors (e.g., financial or family problems) were 5.5 times more likely to have suicidal ideation (Kline et al., 2011). In a study of 275 Iraq and Afghanistan War veterans with subthreshold and threshold PTSD, those reporting subthreshold PTSD were three times more likely to endorse suicidal ideation compared to those without PTSD. In addition, there were no differences in suicidal ideation between the subthreshold and threshold groups, even though—and something that is very relevant for implementing PFA—the subthreshold group was less likely to report prior mental health treatment (Jakupcak et al., 2011). Suicide rates for male veterans between the ages of 18 and 29 years spiked nearly 44% between 2009 and 2011 (Thomas, 2014), and statistics from 2012 indicated that 22 veterans died by suicide per day (Kemp & Bossarte, 2013). The daily veteran suicide rate in 2018 was 17.6, up only slightly from 17.5 per day in 2017, and after adjusting for age and sex, the suicide rate per 100,000 veterans in 2018 was 27.5 (US Department of Veterans Affairs, 2020). To place this in context, the rate of suicide among the general population of the United States was 14.5 per 100,000 in 2019 (Centers for Disease Control and Prevention, 2021).

Factors That Increase Severity

In addition to recognizing the symptoms of normal and potentially more dysfunctional reactions and responses, it is worthwhile to review some of the factors in the literature purported to increase the risk for negative symptoms and symptom severity following a disaster. These factors, some of which might be associated with the individual and others related to the event, might be particularly relevant for PFA providers to familiarize themselves with when they assess an individual to determine his or her disposition.

For first responders, events involving children, occupational stress, a shortage of supplies and resources, a lack of perceived social support, and sleep disturbances have been predictors of psychological symptoms following trauma exposure (Chen et al., 2007; Declercq et al., 2011). Responders with perceived low social support combined with high self-blame following an event were particularly vulnerable to clinical symptoms (Meyer et al., 2012). In a sample of veterans, higher levels of general self-efficacy (confidence in one's ability to produce a desired outcome) have been associated with lower PTSD and depressive symptom severity (Blackburn & Owens, 2015). To support this contention, a study of 245 students enrolled at Virginia Tech at the time of the April 16, 2007, shootings found that posttraumatic stress led to more severe grief reactions due to an undermining of self-efficacy and disruption of one's worldview (i.e., one's sense of meaning and justice in the world) (Smith et al., 2015).

In a study of Manhattan residents following the 9/11 attacks, respondents who acknowledged experiencing severe stressors in the year before the attacks were more likely to have symptoms for both PTSD and depression. Moreover, low levels of social support, the loss of a friend or a relative in the attacks, and the loss of a job due to the attacks were all factors associated with symptoms of depression (Galea et al., 2002). In a sample of veterans residing in the Gulf Coast during Hurricane Katrina, those with preexisting PTSD were 11.9 times more likely to screen positive for any new mental illness (Sullivan et al., 2013).

In a 30-year longitudinal study in a sample of 754 participants, religious service attendance, including more frequent attendance, was shown to correlate significantly with reduced depressive symptoms, while controlling for demographic factors, lifetime trauma, socioeconomic status, and recent negative events (Zou et al., 2014). In a unique study of Islamic-based appraisals in 110 children ages 7 to 13 years old five years after the 2004 tsunami, it was found that the greatest variance (17.1%) in PTSD severity was explained by the belief that being more religious (i.e., honoring Allah) would protect them from future harmful events (Dawson et al., 2014).

In a study of 753 women described as living in an urban Michigan county, physical partner violence within the past 12 months predicted five times higher rates of depression, GAD, PTSD, drug dependence, and alcohol dependence than women who never experienced domestic violence (Tolman & Rosen, 2001). In the aftermath of the 2004 Indian Ocean tsunami, posttrauma mental health difficulties were associated with women (Frankenberg et al., 2008); low-income households (Kumar et al., 2007); lower education levels (Suar, Das, & Hota, 2010); and loss of family members, witnessing the tsunami, or sustaining an injury (Gunaratne et al., 2014). In a sample of 441 police and firefighters from Biloxi and Gulfport, Mississippi, who were involved in the relief efforts following Hurricane Katrina and assessed two years after the hurricane, 18.8% reported having experienced physical victimization before age 18 years, and this was associated with symptoms of PTSD, peritraumatic dissociation, depressive symptoms, and sleep problems (Komarovskaya et al., 2014). In a sample of 145 OEF/OIF veterans, PTSD-depression symptoms had minimal to almost no effect on suicidal ideation when postdeployment social support (receiving tangible resources or support from family, friends, or community) was high; however, when postdeployment social support was low, PTSD-depression symptoms were positively associated with suicidal ideation (DeBeer et al., 2014). As alluded to previously, loneliness due to the need for social distancing and isolation is a signature feature of the COVID-19 pandemic. In fact, in a sample of 1,013 US adults assessed in April 2020, 43% scored above cutoff scores on a loneliness scale (Killgore et al., 2020). These feelings of loneliness were associated with depression and suicidal ideation, and as noted by Czeisler et al. (2020), serious consideration of suicide in the past 30 days in June 2020 was more than twice as high as it was during the previous 12-month reference period (10.7% versus 4.3%). Last, and poignantly, in a study of 381 men and women living in two geographic areas that had differing levels of radiation contamination within Belarus after the Chernobyl incident, Beehler et al. (2008) stated, "In summary, it is noteworthy that almost 20 years after the disaster, psychological distress in Belarusians is better predicted by factors such as mastery/controllability, degree of chronic stressors and perceived family problems than residential radiation exposure" (p. 1248).

This chapter has focused on the unique context of disaster. Disasters, by definition, are overwhelming. Setting expectations for the nature and magnitude of mental health surge can serve to better prepare all disaster responders but especially those applying PFA. Let us review the main points of the chapter:

1. A comprehensive review of data from 284 reports of disaster-related PTSD symptoms published between 1980 and 2008 revealed that the prevalence of PTSD is generally lower after natural disasters compared with human-made and technological disasters (Neria, Nandi, & Galea, 2008).

2. Natural disasters occur because of weather and geological events. The degree of destruction they wreak depends on a variety of factors, including the intensity of the event, the population density where the events occur, and the degree of preparation available, including architectural strength and established warning systems. Natural disasters are often thought to occur at random, though some regions are more prone to certain types of natural disasters. We looked closely at the psychological impacts of Hurricanes Andrew, Katrina, and Sandy, as well as the 2004 Indian Ocean tsunami, the 2008 earthquake in China, the 2010 earthquake in Haiti, the 2011 earthquake and tsunami in Japan, and the COVID-19 pandemic.

3. Technological disasters are defined as events caused by human beings but without intent to harm. This is an important distinction because intention appears to increase psychological toxicity. The psychological impacts of such technological disasters as Three Mile Island, the Chernobyl nuclear accident, the *Exxon Valdez* oil spill, the *Deepwater Horizon* disaster and subsequent oil spill, and

the nuclear plant explosions as a result of the 2011 earthquake and tsunami in Japan are weighed here.

4. In contrast to technological disasters, human-made events are defined by the element of intent to harm and include the sarin gas attacks in Tokyo, the Oklahoma City bombing, the September 11 attacks, the Virginia Tech shooting, the Boston Marathon bombing, and other mass shootings, all reviewed herein. Intention to harm not only adds to psychological toxicity but also seems to contribute to psychological malignancy (catastrophic thought) and contagion.

5. The psychological impact of war, with an emphasis on Operation Iraqi Freedom and Operation Enduring Freedom, include accompanying concerns about traumatic brain injuries and suicide. The fact that within the United States there are many returning veterans suffering from PTSD, traumatic brain injury, and depression suggests the potential for a significant public health challenge in the form of a surge in demand for community mental health services. PFA-trained community mental health professionals and volunteers may serve an important role in expanding mental health surge capacity. Use of PFA-trained volunteers, first responders, and first receivers could do much to address the public health challenge underscored by the Institute of Medicine.

6. Finally, there are data to suggest that certain factors might increase or decrease symptom expression or severity, such as social support, self-efficacy, previous or concurrent stressors, religion, and preexisting diagnoses. These factors are important for PFA interventionists to consider as they formulate intervention and follow-up plans.

References

American Psychiatric Association. (1980). *Diagnostic and statistical manual of mental disorders* (3rd ed.). Washington, DC: American Psychiatric Association.

American Psychiatric Association. (1987). *Diagnostic and statistical manual of mental disorders* (3rd ed., revised). Washington, DC: American Psychiatric Association.

Asukai, N. (1999). *Mental health effects following man-made toxic disasters: The sarin attack and arsenic poisoning case.* Paper presented at the 11th Congress of World Association for Disaster and Emergency Medicine, Osaka, Japan.

Beehler, G. P., Baker, J. A., Falkner, K., Chegerova, T., Pryshchepava, A., Chegerov, V., . . . Moysich, K. B. (2008). A multilevel analysis of long-term psychological distress among Belarusians affected by the Chernobyl disaster. *Public Health, 122,* 1239–1249. http://dx.doi.org/10.1016/j.puhe .2008.04.017.

Ben-Ezra, M., Shigemura, J., Palgi, Y., Hamama-Raz, Y., Lavenda, O., Suzuki, M., & Goodwin, R. (2015). From Hiroshima to Fukushima: PTSD symptoms and radiation stigma across regions in Japan. *Journal of Psychiatric Research, 60,* 185–186. http://dx.doi.org/10.1016/j.jpsychires.2014.10.006.

Blackburn, L., & Owens, G. P. (2015). The effect of self-efficacy and meaning in life on posttraumatic stress disorder and depression severity among veterans. *Journal of Clinical Psychology, 71,* 219–228. http://dx.doi.org/10 .1002/jclp.22133.

Boscarino, J. A., Hoffman, S. N., Kirchner, H. L., Erlich, P. M., Adams, R. E., Figley, C. R., & Solhkhah, R. (2013). Mental health outcomes at the Jersey Shore after Hurricane Sandy. *International Journal of Emergency Mental Health and Human Resilience, 15,* 147–158.

Bowler, R. M., Murai, K., & True, R. H. (2001). Update and long-term sequelae of the sarin attack in the Tokyo, Japan subway. *Chemical Health and Safety, 8,* 53–55.

Brackbill, R. M., Hadler, J. L., DiGrande, L., Ekenga, C. C., Farfel, M. R., Friedman, S., & Thorpe, L. E. (2009). Asthma and posttraumatic stress symptoms 5 to 6 years following exposure to the World Trade Center terrorist attack. *JAMA, 302,* 502–516. http://dx.doi.org/10.1001/jama.2009 .1121.

Bromet, E. J., Havenaar, J. M., & Guey, L. T. (2011). A 25-year retrospective review of the psychological consequences of the Chernobyl accident. *Clinical Oncology, 23,* 297–305. http://dx.doi.org/10.1016/j.clon.2011.01.501.

Bryan, C. J., & Clemans, T. A. (2013). Repetitive traumatic brain injury, psychological symptoms, and suicide risk in a clinical sample of deployed military personnel. *JAMA Psychiatry, 70,* 686–691. http://dx.doi.org/10.1001 /jamapsychiatry.2013.1093.

Caramanica, K., Brackbill, R. M., Liao, T., & Stellman, S. D. (2014). Comorbidity of 9/11-related PTSD and depression in the World Trade Center Health Registry 10–11 years postdisaster. *Journal of Traumatic Stress, 27,* 680–688. http://dx.doi.org/10.1002/jts.21972.

Cénat, J. M., Blais-Rochette, C., Kokou-Kpolou, C. K., Noorishad, P-G., Mukunzi, J. N., McIntee, S-E., ... Labelle, P. R. (2021). Prevalence of symptoms of depression, anxiety, insomnia, posttraumatic stress disorder, and psychological distress among populations affected by the COVID-19 pandemic: A systematic review and meta-analysis. *Psychiatry Research, 295*, 113599. http://dx.doi.org/10.1016/j.psychres.2020.113599.

Center for Human Rights and Global Justice. (2011). *Sexual violence in Haiti's IDP camps: Results of a household survey.* https://chrgj.org/wp-content /uploads/2011/03/HaitiSexualViolenceMarch2011.pdf.

Centers for Disease Control and Prevention. (2021). *Suicide and self-inflicted injury.* Retrieved on August 27, 2021, from http://www.cdc.gov /nchs/fastats/suicide.htm.

Cerdá, M., Paczkowski, M., Galea, S., Nemethy, K., Péan, C., & Desvarieux, M. (2013). Psychopathology in the aftermath of the Haiti earthquake: A population-based study of posttraumatic stress disorder and major depression. *Depression and Anxiety, 30*, 413–424. http://dx.doi.org/10.1002 /da.22007.

Chen, Y. S., Chen, M. C., Chou, F. H., Sun, F. C., Chen, P. C., Tsai, K. Y., & Chao, S. S. (2007). The relationship between quality of life and posttraumatic stress disorder or major depression for firefighters in Kaohsiung, Taiwan. *Quality of Life Research, 16*, 1289–1297. http://dx.doi.org/10.1007 /s11136-007-9248-7.

Cleary, P. D., & Houts, P. S. (1984). The psychological impact of the Three Mile Island incident. *Journal of Human Stress, 10*, 28–34. http://dx.doi.org /10.1080/0097840X.1984.9934956.

Clemens, P., Hietala, J. R., Rytter, M. J., Schmidt, R. A., & Reese, D. J. (1999). Risk of domestic violence after flood impacts: Effects of social support, age and history of domestic violence. *Applied Behavioral Science Review, 7*, 199–206. http://dx.doi.org/10.1016/S1068-8595(00)80020-3.

CNN Editorial Research. (2021). Hurricane Katrina statistics fast facts. *CNN Weather.* Retrieved on August 27, 2021, from https://edition.cnn.com/2013 /08/23/us/hurricane-Katrina-statistics-fast-facts/index.html.

Curtis, T., Miller, B. C., & Berry, E. H. (2000). Changes in reports and incidence of child abuse following natural disasters. *Child Abuse & Neglect, 24*, 1151–1162. http://dx.doi.org/10.1016/S0145-2134(00)00176-9.

Cutler, D. M., & Summers, L. H. (2020). The COVID-19 pandemic and the $16 trillion virus. *JAMA, 324*, 1495–1496. http://dx.doi.org/10.1001/jama .2020.19759.

Czeisler, M. É., Lane, R. I., Petrosky, E., Wiley, J. F., Christensen, A., Njai, R., ... Rajaratnam, S. M. W. (2020). Mental health, substance use, and sui-

cidal ideation during the COVID-19 pandemic—United States, June 24–
30, 2020. *Morbidity and Mortality Weekly Report (MMWR), 69*, 1049–1057.
http://dx.doi.org/10.15585/mmwr.mm6932a1.

David, D., Mellman, T. A., Mendoza, L. M., Kulick-Bell, R., Ironson, G., &
Schneiderman, N. (1996). Psychiatric morbidity following Hurricane
Andrew. *Journal of Traumatic Stress, 9*, 607–612. http://dx.doi.org/10
.1007/BF02103669.

Davidson, L. M., & Baum, A. (1986). Chronic stress and post-traumatic stress
disorders. *Journal of Consulting and Clinical Psychology, 33*, 303–308. http://dx
.doi.org/10.1037/0022-006X.54.3.303.

Dawson, K. S., Joscelyne, A., Meijer, C., Tampubolon, A., Steel, Z., & Bryant,
R. A. (2014). Predictors of chronic posttraumatic response in Muslim chil-
dren following natural disasters. *Psychological Trauma: Theory, Research,
Practice, and Policy, 6*, 580–587. http://dx.doi.org/10.1037/a0037140.

DeBeer, B. B., Kimbrel, N. A., Meyer, E. C., Gulliver, S. B., & Morissette, S. B.
(2014). Combined PTSD and depressive symptoms interact with postdeployment social support to predict suicidal ideation in Operation
Enduring Freedom and Operation Iraqi Freedom veterans. *Psychiatry
Research, 216*, 357–362. http://dx.doi.org/10.1016/j.psychres.2014.02.010.

Declercq, F., Maganck, R., Deheegher, J., & Van Hoorde, H., (2011). Frequency
of and subjective response to critical incidents in the prediction of PTSD
in emergency personnel. *Journal of Traumatic Stress, 24*, 133–136. http://dx
.doi.org/10.1002/jts.20609.

DeMartino, R. (2002, November 19). *Bio-terrorism: What are we afraid of and
what should we do.* Paper presented at the Biosecurity 2002 Conference,
Las Vegas, NV.

Deryugina, T., Kawano, L., & Levitt, S. (2018). The economic impact of Hurricane Katrina on its victims: Evidence from individual tax returns. *American Economic Journal: Applied Economics, 10*, 202–233. http://dx.doi.org/10
.1257/app.20160307.

Dew, M. A., & Bromet, E. J. (1993). Predictors of temporal patterns of psychiatric distress during 10 years following the nuclear accident at Three Mile
Island. *Social Psychiatry and Psychiatric Epidemiology, 28*, 49–55. http://dx
.doi.org/10.1007/BF00802091.

Drescher, C. F., Schulenberg, S. E., & Smith, C. V. (2014). The *Deepwater Horizon* oil spill and the Mississippi Gulf Coast: Mental health in the context
of a technological disaster. *American Journal of Orthopsychiatry, 84*, 142–
151. http://dx.doi.org/10.1037/h0099382.

Du, J., Dong, L., Wang, T., Yuan, C., Fu, R., Zhang, L., . . . Li, X. (2020). Psychological symptoms among frontline healthcare workers during COVID-19

outbreak in Wuhan. *General Hospital Psychiatry, 67*, 144–145. http://dx.doi
.org/10.1016/j.genhosppsych.2020.03.011.

Everytown for Gun Safety Support Fund. (2021). *Twelve years of mass
shootings in the United States: An Everytown for Gun Safety Support Fund
analysis.* Everytown Research and Policy, last updated June 4, 2021. https:
//everytownresearch.org/maps/mass-shootings-in-america-2009–2019.

Foster, R. P., & Goldstein, M. F. (2007). Chernobyl disaster sequelae in recent
immigrants to the United States from the former Soviet Union (FSU).
Journal of Immigrant and Minority Health, 9, 115–124. http://dx.doi.org/10
.1007/s10903-006-9024-8.

Frankenberg, E., Friedman, J., Gillespie, T., Ingwersen, N., Pynoos, R.,
Rifai, I. U., . . . Duncan, T. (2008). Mental health in Sumatra after the
tsunami. *American Journal of Public Health, 98*, 1671–1677. http://dx.doi
.org/10.2105/AJPH.2007.120915.

Friedland, N., & Merari, A. (1985). The psychological impact of terrorism:
A double-edged sword. *Political Psychology, 6*, 591–604. http://dx.doi.org
/10.2307/3791018.

Galea, S., Ahern, J., Resnick, H., Kilpatrick, D., Bucuvalas, M., Gold, J., &
Vlahov, D. (2002). Psychological sequelae of the September 11 terrorist
attacks in New York City. *New England Journal of Medicine, 346*, 982–987.
http://dx.doi.org/10.1056/NEJMsa013404.

Galea, S., Brewin, C. R., Gruber, M., Jones, R. T., King, D. W., King, L. A., &
Kessler, R. C. (2007). Exposure to hurricane-related stressors and mental
illness after Hurricane Katrina. *Archives of General Psychiatry, 64*, 1427–1434.
http://dx.doi.org/10.1001/archpsyc.64.12.1427.

Gates, J. D., Arabian, S., Biddinger, P., Blansfield, J., Burke, P., Chung, S., . . .
Yaffe, M. B. (2014). The initial response to the Boston Marathon bombing:
Lessons learned to prepare for the next disaster. *Annals of Surgery, 260*,
960–966. http://dx.doi.org/10.1097/SLA.0000000000000914.

Gill, D. A., Picou, J. S., & Ritchie, L. A. (2011). The *Exxon Valdez* and BP oil
spills: A comparison of initial social and psychological impacts. *American
Behavioral Scientist, 56*, 3–23. http://dx.doi.org/10.1177/0002764211408585.

Grattan, L. M., Roberts, S., Mahan, W. T., Jr., McLaughlin, P. K., Otwell, W. S.,
& Morris, J. G. (2011). The early psychological impacts of the *Deepwater
Horizon* oil spill on Florida and Alabama communities. *Environmental
Health Perspectives, 119*, 839–843. http://dx.doi.org/10.1289/ehp.1002915.

Gunaratne, C., Kremer, P. J., Clarke, V., & Lewis, A. J. (2014). Trauma-related
symptoms in Sri Lankan adult survivors after the Tsunami: Pretrauma and
peritrauma factors. *Asia-Pacific Journal of Public Health, 26*, 425–434.
http://dx.doi.org/10.1177/1010539513500337.

Haitian Conference, Government of the Republic of Haiti. (2010, March). *Action plan for national recovery and development of Haiti: Immediate key initiatives for the future.* https://www.recoveryplatform.org/assets/publication /Action_Plan_12April_haiti.pdf.

Havenaar, J. M., Rumyantzeva, G. M., van den Brink, W., Poelijoe, N. W., van den Bout, J., van Engeland, H., & Koeter, M. W. J. (1997). Long-term mental health effects of the Chernobyl disaster: An epidemiologic survey in two former Soviet regions. *American Journal of Psychiatry, 154,* 1605–1607. http://dx.doi.org/10.1176/ajp.154.11.1605.

History.com Editors. (2018, August 25). *September 11 attacks.* History Channel, last updated August 24, 2021. http://www.history.com/topics/9-11-attacks.

Hoge, C. W., Auchterlonie, J. L., & Milliken, C. S. (2006). Mental health problems, use of mental health services, and attrition from military service after returning from deployment to Iraq or Afghanistan. *JAMA, 295,* 1023–1032. http://dx.doi.org/10.1001/jama.295.9.1023.

Hoge, C. W., Castro, C. A., Messer, S. C., McGurk, D., Cotting, D. I., & Koffman, R. L. (2004). Combat duty in Iraq and Afghanistan, mental health problems, and barriers to care. *New England Journal of Medicine, 351,* 13–22. http://dx.doi.org/10.1056/NEJMoa040603.

Hoge, C. W., McGurk, D., Thomas, J. L., Cox, A. L., Engel, C. C., & Castro, C. A. (2008). Mild traumatic brain injury in US soldiers returning from Iraq. *New England Journal of Medicine, 358,* 453–463. http://dx.doi.org/10.1056 /NEJMoa072972.

Hollifield, M., Hewage, C., Gunawardena, C. N., Kodituwakku, P., Bopagoda, K., & Weerarathnege, K. (2008). Symptoms and coping in Sri Lanka 20–21 months after the 2004 tsunami. *British Journal of Psychiatry, 192,* 39–44. http://dx.doi.org/10.1192/bjp.bp.107.038422.

Holmes, E. A., O'Connor, R. C., Perry, V. H., Tracey, I., Wessely, S., Arseneault, L., … Bullmore, E. (2020). Multidisciplinary research priorities for the COVID-19 pandemic: A call for action for mental health science. *The Lancet Psychiatry, 7,* 547–560. http://dx.doi.org/10.1016/S2215-0366(20)30168-1.

Hughes, M., Brymer, M., Chiu, W. T., Fairbank, J. A., Jones, R. T., Pynoos, R. S., … Steinberg, A. M. (2011). Posttraumatic stress among students after the shootings at Virginia Tech. *Psychological Trauma: Theory, Research, Practice, and Policy, 3,* 403–411. http://dx.doi.org/10.1037/a0024565.

iCasualties. (n.d.). Operation Iraqi Freedom: Iraq coalition military fatalities by year. Retrieved on August 19, 2021, from http://icasualties.org.

Ironson, G., Wynings, C., Schneiderman, N., Baum, A., Rodriguez, M., Greenwood, D., … Fletcher, M. A. (1997). Posttraumatic stress symptoms, intrusive thoughts, loss, and immune function after Hurricane Andrew.

Psychosomatic Medicine, 59, 128–141. http://dx.doi.org/10.1097/00006842 -199703000-00003.

Jakupcak, M., Hoerster, K. D., Varra, A., Vannoy, S., Felker, B., & Hunt, S. (2011). Hopelessness and suicidal ideation in Iraq and Afghanistan War veterans reporting subthreshold and threshold posttraumatic stress disorder. *Journal of Nervous and Mental Disease, 199,* 272–275. http://dx.doi.org /10.1097/NMD.0b013e3182124604.

Johns Hopkins University & Medicine (2022, January 28). Coronavirus Resource Center. https://coronavirus.jhu.edu.

Kawakami, N., Takeshima, T., Ono, Y., Uda, H., Hata, Y., Nakane, Y.,... Kikkawa, T. (2005). Twelve-month prevalence, severity, and treatment of common mental health disorders in communities in Japan: Preliminary finding from the World Mental Health Japan Survey 2002–2003. *Psychiatry and Clinical Neurosciences, 59,* 441–452. http://dx.doi.org/10.1111/j.1440 -1819.2005.01397.x.

Kemp, J., & Bossarte, R. (2013). *Suicide data report, 2012.* Washington, DC: US Department of Veterans Affairs, Mental Health Services.

Kessler, R. C., Galea, S., Gruber, M. J., Sampson, N. A., Ursano, R. J., & Wessely, S. (2008). Trends in mental illness and suicidality after Hurricane Katrina. *Molecular Psychiatry, 13,* 374–384. http://dx.doi.org/10.1038/sj .mp.4002119.

Killgore, W. D. S., Cloonan, S. A., Taylor, E. C., & Dailey, N. S. (2020). Loneliness: A signature mental health concern in the era of COVID-19. *Psychiatry Research, 290,* 113117. http://dx.doi.org/10.1016/j.psychres.2020.113117.

Kline, A., Ciccone, D. S., Falca-Dodson, M., Black, C. M., & Losonczy, M. (2011). Suicidal ideation among National Guard troops deployed to Iraq: The association with postdeployment readjustment problems. *Journal of Nervous and Mental Disease, 199,* 914–920. http://dx.doi.org /10.1097/NMD.0b013e3182392917.

Komarovskaya, I., Brown, A. D., Galatzer-Levy, I. R., Madan, A., Henn-Haase, C., Teater, J.,... Chemtom, C. M. (2014). Early physical victimization is a risk factor for posttraumatic stress disorder symptoms among Mississippi police and firefighter first responders to Hurricane Katrina. *Psychological Trauma: Theory, Research, Practice, and Policy, 6,* 92–96. http://dx.doi .org/10.1037/a0031600.

Kukihara, H., Yamawaki, N., Uchiyama, K., Arai, S., &Horikawa, E. (2014). Trauma, depression, and resilience of earthquake/tsunami/nuclear disaster survivors of Hirono, Fukushima, Japan. *Psychiatry and Clinical Neurosciences, 68,* 524–533. http://dx.doi.org/10.1111/pcn.12159.

Kumar, M. S., Murhekar, M. V., Hutin, Y., Subramanian, T., Ramachandran, V., & Gupte, M. D. (2007). Prevalence of posttraumatic stress disorder in a coastal fishing village in Tamil Nadu, India, after the December 2004 tsunami. *American Journal of Public Health, 97*, 99–101. http://dx.doi.org /10.2105/AJPH.2005.071167.

Lai, J., Ma., S., Wang, Y., Cai, Z., Hu, J., Wei, N., . . . Hu. S. (2020). Factors associated with mental health outcomes among health care workers exposed to coronavirus disease 2019. *JAMA Network Open, 3*, e203976. http://dx.doi .org/10.1001/jamanetworkopen.2020.3976.

Landrigan, P. J., Lioy, P. J., Thurston, G., Berkowitz, G., Chen, L. C., Chillrud, S. N., . . . NIEHS World Trade Center Working Group. (2004). Health and environmental consequences of the World Trade Center disaster. *Environmental Health Perspectives, 112*, 731–739. http://dx.doi.org/10.1289/ehp.6702.

Leander, N. P., Kreienkamp, J., Agostini, M., Stroebe, W., Gordijn, E. H., & Kruglanski, A. W. (2020). Biased hate crime perceptions can reveal supremacist sympathies. *PNAS, 117*, 19072–19079. http://dx.doi.org/10.1073/pnas .1916883117.

LeardMann, C. A., Smith, T. C., Smith, B., Wells, T. S., & Ryan, M. A. K. (2009). Baseline self-reported functional health and vulnerability to posttraumatic stress disorder after combat deployment: Prospective US military cohort study. *BMJ, 338*, b1273. http://dx.doi.org/10.1136/bmj.b1273.

Lei, L., Huang, X., Zhang, S., Yang, J., Yang, L., & Xu, M. (2020). Comparison of prevalence and associated factors of anxiety and depression among people affected by versus people unaffected by quarantine during the COVID-19 epidemic in Southwestern China. *Medical Science Monitor, 26*, e924609-1–e924609-12. http://dx.doi.org/10.12659/msm.924609.

Liu, C. H., Zhang, E., Wong, G. T. F., Hyun, S., & Hahm, H. C. (2020). Factors associated with depression, anxiety, and PTSD symptomatology during the COVID-19 pandemic: Clinical implications for US young adult mental health. *Psychiatry Research, 290*, 113172. http://dx.doi.org/10.1016 /j.psychres.2020.113172.

Loganovsky, K., Havenaar, J. M., Tintle, N. L., Guey, L. T., Kotov, R., & Bromet, E. J. (2008). The mental health of clean-up workers 18 years after the Chernobyl accident. *Psychological Medicine, 38*, 481–488. http://dx.doi.org /10.1017/S0033291707002371.

Lopez, Leo, III, Hart, L. H., III, & Katz, M. H. (2021). Racial and ethnic health disparities related to COVID-19. *JAMA, 325*, 719–720. http://dx.doi.org /10.1001/jama.2020.26443.

Magruder, K. M., & Yeager, D. E. (2009). The prevalence of PTSD across war eras and the effect of deployment on PTSD: A systematic review and meta-analysis. *Psychiatric Annals, 39,* 778–788. http://dx.doi.org/10.3928 /00485713-20090728-04.

Maguen, S., Lucenko, B. A., Reger, M. A., Gahm, G. A., Litz, B. T., Seal, K. H., … Marmar, C. R. (2010). The impact of reported direct and indirect killing on mental health symptoms in Iraq War veterans. *Journal of Traumatic Stress, 23,* 86–90. http://dx.doi.org/10.1002/jts.20434.

Martino, C. (2002). Psychological consequences of terrorism. *International Journal of Emergency Mental Health, 4,* 105–111.

McCartney, M. (2011). Nuclear panic overshadows Japan's real plight. *British Medical Journal, 342,* 686. http://dx.doi.org/10.1136/bmj.d1845.

McLeish, A. C., & Del Ben, K. S. (2008). Symptoms of depression and posttraumatic stress disorder in an outpatient population before and after Hurricane Katrina. *Depression and Anxiety, 25,* 416–421. http://dx.doi.org /10.1002/da.20426.

Meyer, E. C., Zimering, R., Daly, E., Knight, J., Kamholz, B. W., & Gulliver, S. B. (2012). Predictors of posttraumatic stress disorder and other physiological symptoms in trauma-exposed firefighters. *Psychological Services, 9,* 1–15. http://dx.doi.org/10.1037/a0026414.

Miller, M. W., Wolf, E. J., Hein, C., Prince, L., & Reardon, A. F. (2013). Psychological effects of the marathon bombing on Boston-area veterans with posttraumatic stress disorder. *Journal of Traumatic Stress, 26,* 762–766. http://dx.doi.org/10.1002/Jts.21865.

Moghanibashi-Mansourieh, A. (2020). Assessing the anxiety level of Iranian general population during the COVID-19 outbreak. *Asian Journal of Psychiatry, 51,* 102076. http://dx.doi.org/10.1016/j.ajp.2020.102076.

Mong, M., Noguchi, K., & Ladner, B. (2012). Immediate psychological impact of the *Deepwater Horizon* oil spill: Symptoms of PTSD and coping skills. *Journal of Aggression, Maltreatment & Trauma, 21,* 691–704. http://dx.doi.org /10.1080/10926771.2012.694402.

Munich Re. (2021, January 7). Record hurricane season and major wildfires: The natural disaster figures for 2020 [press release]. https://www.muni chre.com/en/company/media-relations/media-information-and-corporate -news/media-information/2021/2020-natural-disasters-balance.html.

Neria, Y., Nandi, A., & Galea, S. (2008). Post-traumatic stress disorder following disasters: A systematic review. *Psychological Medicine, 38,* 467–480. http://dx.doi.org/10.1017/S0033291707001353.

Neria, Y., & Shultz, J. M. (2012). Mental health effects of Hurricane Sandy: Characteristics, potential aftermath, and response. *JAMA, 308,* 2571–2572. http://dx.doi.org/10.1001/jama.2012.110700.

Neuner, F., Shauner, E., Catani, C., Ruf, M., & Elbert, T. (2006). Post-tsunami stress: A study of posttraumtic stress disorder in children living in three severely affected regions in Sri Lanka. *Journal of Traumatic Stress, 19*, 339–347. http://dx.doi.org/10.1002/jts.20121.

Norris, F. H., Friedman, M. J., Watson, P. J., Byrne, C. M., Diaz, E., & Kaniasty, K. (2002). 60,000 disaster victims speak: Part I. An empirical review of the empirical literature, 1981–2001. *Psychiatry: Interpersonal and Biological Processes, 65*, 207–239. http://dx.doi.org/10.1521/psyc.65.3.207.20173.

North, C. S., Nixon, S. J., Shariat, S., Mallonee, S., McMillen, C., Spitznagel, E. L., & Smith, E. M. (1999). Psychiatric disorders among survivors of the Oklahoma City bombing. *JAMA, 282*, 755–762. http://dx.doi.org/10.1001/jama.282.8.755.

North, C. S., Tivis, L., McMillen, J. C., Pfefferbaum, B., Spitznagel, E. L., Cox, J.,... Smith, E. M. (2002). Psychiatric disorders in rescue workers after the Oklahoma City bombing. *American Journal of Psychiatry, 159*, 857–859. http://dx.doi.org/10.1176/appi.ajp.159.5.857.

Ohbu, S., Yamashina, A., Takasu, N., Yamaguchi, T., Murai, T., Nakano, K.,... Hinohara, S. (1997). Sarin poisoning on Tokyo subway. *Southern Medical Journal, 90*, 587–593. http://doi.org/10.1097/00007611-199706000-00002.

Palgi, Y., Ben-Ezra, M., Aviel, O., Dubiner, Y., Baruch, E., Soffer, Y., & Shrira, A. (2012). Mental health and disaster related attitudes among Japanese after the 2011 Fukushima nuclear disaster [letter to the editor]. *Journal of Psychiatric Research, 46*, 688–690. http://dx.doi.org/10.1016/j.jpsychires.2012.01.028.

Palinkas, L. A., Petterson, J. S., Russell, J., & Downs, M. A. (1993). Community patterns of psychiatric disorders after the *Exxon Valdez* oil spill. *American Journal of Psychiatry, 150*, 1517–1523. http://dx.doi.org/10.1176/ajp.150.10.1517.

Pappa, S., Ntella, V., Giannakas, T., Giannakoulis, V. G., Papoutsi, E., & Katsaounou, P. (2020). Prevalence of depression, anxiety, and insomnia among healthcare workers during the COVID-19 pandemic: A systematic review and meta-analysis. *Brain, Behavior, and Immunity, 88*, 901–907. http://dx.doi.org/10.1016/j.bbi.2020.05.026.

Perlman, S. E., Friedman, S., Galea, S., Nair, H. P., Erós-Sarnyai, M., Stellman, S. D.,... Greene, C. M. (2011). Short-term and medium-term health effects of 9/11. *The Lancet, 378*, 925–934. http://dx.doi.org/10.1016/S0140-6736(11)60967-7.

Perrin, M. A., DiGrande, L., Wheeler, K., Thorpe, L., Farfel, M., & Brackbill, R. (2007). Differences in PTSD prevalence and associated risk factors among World Trade Center disaster rescue and recovery workers. *Ameri-*

can *Journal of Psychiatry, 164*, 1385–1394. http://dx.doi.org/10.1176/appi.ajp
.2007.06101645.

Phillips, C. J., LeardMann, C. A., Gumbs, G. R., & Smith, B. (2010). Risk factors for posttraumatic stress disorder among deployed US male marines. *BMC Psychiatry, 10*, 52. http://dx.doi.org/10.1186/1471-244X-10-52.

Prince-Embury, S., & Rooney, J. F. (1988). Psychological symptoms of residents in the aftermath of the Three Mile Island nuclear accident and restart. *Journal of Social Psychology, 128*, 779–790. http://dx.doi.org/10.1080/00224545.1988.9924556.

Propper, R. E., Stickgold, R., Keeley, R., & Christman, S. D., (2007). Is television traumatic? Dreams, stress and media exposure in the aftermath of September 11, 2001. *Psychological Science, 18*, 334–340. http://dx.doi.org/10.1111/j.1467-9280.2007.01900.x.

Rahill, G. J., Joshi, M., Lescano, C., & Holbert, D. (2015). Symptoms of PTSD in a sample of female victims of sexual violence in post-earthquake Haiti. *Journal of Affective Disorders, 173*, 232–238. http://dx.doi.org/10.1016/j.jad.2014.10.067.

Rashid, S. F. (2000). The urban poor in Dhaka City: Their struggles and coping strategies during the floods of 1998. *Disasters, 24*, 240–253. http://dx.doi.org/10.1111/1467-7717.00145.

Richman, J. A., Shannon, C. A., Rospenda, K. M., Flaherty, J. A., & Fendrich, M. (2009). The relationship between terrorism and distress and drinking: Two years after September 11, 2001. *Substance Use & Misuse, 44*, 1665–1680. http://dx.doi.org/10.3109/10826080902961989.

Robertson, C., & Krauss, C. (2010, August 3). Gulf spill is the largest of its kind, scientists say. *New York Times*, p. A14.

Rosenbaum, S. (2006). US health policy in the aftermath of Hurricane Katrina. *JAMA, 295*, 437–440. http://dx.doi.org/10.1001/jama.295.4.437.

Rosenberg, J. (2014). Mass shootings and mental health policy. *Journal of Sociology & Social Welfare, 16*, 107–121.

Sakuma, A., Takahashi, Y., Ueda, I., Sato, H., Katsura, M. Abe, . . . Matsumoto, K. (2015). Post-traumatic stress disorder and depression prevalence and associated risk factors among local disaster relief and reconstruction workers fourteen months after the Great East Japan Earthquake: A cross-sectional study. *BioMed Central Psychiatry, 15*, 58. http://dx.doi.org/10.1186/s12888-015-0440-y.

Schlenger, W. E., Caddell, J. M., Ebert, L., Jordan, K. B., Rourke, K. M., Wilson, D., . . . Kulka, R. A. (2002). Psychological reactions to terrorist attacks: Findings from the national study of Americans' reactions to September 11. *JAMA, 288*, 581–588. http://dx.doi.org/10.1001/jama.288.5.581.

Shariat, S., Mallonee, S., Kruger, E., Farmer, K., & North, C. (1999). A prospective study of long-term health outcomes among Oklahoma City bombing survivors. *Journal of the Oklahoma State Medical Association, 92,* 178–186.

Shenesey, J. W., & Langhinrichsen-Rohling, J. (2015). Perceived resilience: Examining impacts of the *Deepwater Horizon* oil spill one-year post-spill. *Psychological Trauma: Theory, Research, Practice, and Policy, 7,* 252–258. http://dx.doi.org/10.1037/a0035182.

Shigemura, J., Tanigawa, T., Saito, I., & Nomura, S. (2012). Psychological distress in workers at the Fukushima nuclear power plants. *JAMA, 308,* 667–669. http://dx.doi.org/10.1001/jama.2012.9699.

Smith, A. J., Abeyta, A. A., Hughes, M., & Jones, R. T. (2015). Persistent grief in the aftermath of mass violence: The predictive roles of posttraumatic stress symptoms, self-efficacy, and disrupted worldview. *Psychological Trauma: Theory, Research, Practice and Policy, 7,* 179–186. http://dx.doi.org /10.1037/tra0000002.

Statista. (2021, February 2). *Annual number of natural disaster events globally from 2000 to 2020.* https://www.statista.com/statistics/510959/number-of -natural-disasters-events-globally.

Stellman, J. M., Smith, R. P., Katz, C. L., Sharma, V., Charney, D. S. Herbert, R., ... Southwick, S. (2008). Enduring mental health morbidity and social function impairment in World Trade Center rescue, recovery, and cleanup workers: The psychological dimension of an environmental health disaster. *Environmental Health Perspective, 116,* 1248–1253. http://dx.doi.org/10 .1289/ehp.11164.

Suar, D., Das, N., & Hota, L. B. (2010). Social indicators affecting post-tsunami trauma survivors. *Journal of Health Management, 12,* 483–500. http://doi.org/10.1177/097206341001200405.

Sullivan, G., Vasterling, J. J., Han, X., Tharp, A. T., Davis, T., Deitch, E. A., & Constans, J. I. (2013). Preexisting mental illness and risk for developing a new disorder after Hurricane Katrina. *Journal of Nervous and Mental Disease, 201,* 161–166. http://dx.doi.org/10.1097/NMD.0b013e31827 f636d.

Talbott, E. O., Youk, A. O., McHugh-Pemu, K. P., & Zborowski, J. V. (2003). Long-term follow-up of the residents of the Three Mile Island accident area: 1979–1998. *Environmental Health Perspectives, 111,* 341–348. http://dx.doi .org/10.1289/ehp.5662.

Telford, J., Cosgrave, J., & Houghton, R. (2006). *Joint evaluation of the international response to the Indian Ocean tsunami: Synthesis report.* London, England: Tsunami Evaluation Coalition.

Thomas, E. (2014, January 1). Suicide among young veterans rising at alarming rate. *Huffington Post.* http://www.huffingtonpost.com/2014/01/10/young-veteran-suicide-doubles_n_4576846.html.

Tolman, R. M., & Rosen, D. (2001). Domestic violence in the lives of women receiving welfare: Mental health, substance dependence, and economic well-being. *Violence against Women, 7,* 141–158. http://dx.doi.org/10.1177/1077801201007002003.

Tone, M., & Stone, T. (2014). What we can learn about recovery: Lessons from the Fukushima survivors. *Nursing Health Science, 16,* 52–55. http://dx.doi.org/10.1111/nhs.12117.

Tucker, P., Dickson, W., Pfefferbaum, B., McDonald, N. B., & Allen, G. (1997). Traumatic reactions as predictors of posttraumatic stress six months after the Oklahoma City bombing. *Psychiatric Services, 48,* 1191–1194.

Ursano, R. J., Norwood, A. E., Fullerton, C. S., Holloway, H. C., & Hall, M. (2003). Terrorism with weapons of mass destruction: Chemical, biological, nuclear, radiological, and explosive agents. In R. J. Ursano and A. E. Norwood (Eds.), *Trauma and disaster: Responses and management* (pp. 125–154). Washington, DC: American Psychiatric Publishing.

US Department of Defense. (n.d.). *Casualty status: Operation Iraqi Freedom U.S. casualty status* [table]. Retrieved on August 19, 2021 from http://www.defense.gov/casualty.pdf.

US Department of Veterans Affairs, Office of Mental Health and Suicide Prevention. (2020). *2020 National Veteran Suicide Prevention annual report.* Washington, DC: Department of Veterans Affairs. http://www.mentalhealth.va.gov/docs/data-sheets/2020/2020-National-Veteran-Suicide-Prevention-Annual-Report-11-2020-508.pdf.

Vasterling, J. J., Brailey, K., Proctor, S. P., Kane, R., Heeren, T., & Franz, M. (2012). Neuropsychological outcomes of mild traumatic brain injury, post-traumatic disorder and depression in Iraq-deployed US Army soldiers. *British Journal of Psychiatry, 201,* 186- 192. http://dx.doi.org/10.1192/bjp.bp.111.096461.

Velavan, T. P., & Meyer, C. G. (2020). The COVID-19 epidemic. *Tropical Medicine & International Health, 25,* 278–280. http://dx.doi.org/10.1111/tmi.13383.

Walsh, W. M., & Schwartz, N. D. (2012, November 1). Estimate of economic losses now up to $50 billion. *New York Times.* http://www.nytimes.com/2012/11/02/business/estimate-of-economic-losses-now-up-to-50-billion.html.

Watson Institute International & Public Affairs (2020, January). *Economic costs.* Costs of War. https://watson.brown.edu/costsofwar/costs/economic.

Watts, J. (1999). Tokyo terrorist attacks: Effects still felt 4 years on. *The Lancet, 353*, 569. http://dx.doi.org/10.1016/S0140-6736(05)75637-3.

Welch, A. E., Caramanica, K., Maslow, C. B., Cone, J. E., Farfel, M. R., Keyes, K. M.,... Hasin, D. S. (2014). Frequent binge drinking five to six years after exposure to 9/11: Findings from the World Trade Center Health Registry. *Drug and Alcohol Dependence, 140*, 1–7. http://dx.doi.org/10.1016/j.drugalcdep .2014.04.013.

West, C., Bernard, B., Mueller, C., Kitt, M., Driscoll, R., & Sangwoo, T. (2008). Mental health outcomes in police personnel after Hurricane Katrina. *Journal of Occupational and Environmental Medicine, 50*, 689–695. http://dx.doi .org/10.1097/JOM.0b013e3181638685.

Wickrama, K. A., & Kaspar, V. (2007). Family context of mental health risk in tsunami-exposed adolescents: Findings from a pilot study in Sri Lanka. *Social Science and Medicine, 64*, 713–723. http://dx.doi.org/10.1016/j.socsci med.2006.09.031.

Wiersinga, W. J., & Prescott, H. C. (2020). What is COVID-19? *JAMA, 324*, 816. http://dx.doi.org/10.1001/jama.2020.12984.

Willman, A., & Marcelin, L. H. (2010). If they could make it disappear, they would: Youth and violence in Cité Soleil, Haiti. *Journal of Community Psychology, 38*, 515–531. http://dx.doi.org/10.1002/jcop.20379.

Wiseman, H., Metzl, E., & Barber, J. L. (2006). Anger, guilt, and intergenerational communication of trauma in the interpersonal narratives of second generation Holocaust survivors. *American Journal of Orthopsychiatry, 78*, 176–184. http://dx.doi.org/10.1037/0002-9432.76.2.176.

Xu, J., Mo, L., & Wu, Z. (2013). A cross-sectional study on risk factors of depression severity among survivors of the 2008 Sichuan Earthquake. *Community Mental Health Journal, 49*, 847–856. http://dx.doi.org/10.1007 /s10597-012-9578-y.

Yehuda, R., Bell, A., Bierer, L. M., & Schmeidler, J. (2008). Maternal, not paternal, PTSD, is related to increased risk for PTSD in offspring of Holocaust survivors. *Journal of Psychiatric Research, 42*, 1104–1111. http://dx .doi.org/10.1016/j.jpsychires.2008.01.002.

Yin, Q., Chen, A., Song, X., Deng, G., & Dong, W. (2021). Risk perception and PTSD symptoms of medical staff combating against COVID-19: A PLS structural equation model. *Frontiers in Psychiatry, 12*, 607612. http://dx.doi .org/10.3389/fpsyt.2021.607612.

Zou, J., Huang, Y., Maldonado, L., Kasen, S., Cohen, P., & Chen, H. (2014). The efficacy of religious service attendance in reducing depressive symptoms. *Social Psychiatry and Psychiatric Epidemiology, 49*, 911–918. http://dx .doi.org/10.1007/s00127-013-0785-9.

PSYCHOLOGICAL FIRST AID

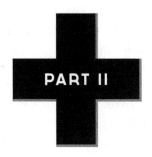

PART II

PRACTICING THE ART

In this second part of the book, we explain the Johns Hopkins RAPID model of PFA in step-by-step fashion while using an integrating pre-COVID-19 scenario to provide an ongoing example of how RAPID may be applied and how it might actually sound. Remember from chapter 1 that RAPID is an acronym that denotes the model's constituent phases:

R—Rapport and reflective listening. Effective psychological crisis intervention is predicated upon gaining rapport with the person in distress. Rapport may be thought of as a form of interpersonal "connectedness" that serves as a platform for the remaining aspects of the model.

A—Assessment. The term *assessment* is used liberally here and consists of screening (Is there any evidence of need for PFA or other types of intervention?) and appraisal (What is the severity or gravity of need?). This information is generated not through the use of psychological tests or mental status examinations but instead through listening to the person's story of distress. The story consists of what happened (the stressor event) and the person's reactions (signs and symptoms) in response to the event.

P—Prioritization. Having heard the story, you must determine whether the need for intervention is urgent. This becomes an exercise in psychological triage.

I—Intervention. Having heard the story and the associated reactions, making some effort to stabilize and mitigate the adverse reactions is often recommended, if not expected.

D—Disposition. Having heard the story and responded with an appropriate intervention, you now must determine what to do next. "Where do we go from here?" is a question you should ask yourself and might even ask the person you've assisted. Is the person capable of attending to his or her responsibilities or is a referral to some higher level of care indicated?

FIVE

R—Rapport and
Reflective Listening

Establishing a Relationship

> Prophylactically, it is probable that many
> disorders could be nipped in the bud if prompt
> attention could be given to germinating seeds
> which may later grow into tall oaks.
>
> —F. C. THORNE, discussing the
> foundations of psychological first aid

ESTABLISHING SOME DEGREE of *rapport* is the first objective for the psychological first aid (PFA) provider. Rapport may be thought of as some degree of interpersonal connectedness, understanding, and even trust.

First Things First:
The Practice of Presence

Rapport begins with presence. Rapport is built on the perception of the present interventionist (i.e., having a physical and/ or emotional presence) and is sometimes what the person in distress needs most. Many care providers have referred to this as a *ministry of presence*. Ministry does not refer to a religious presence but, rather, to caring attention for another person.

Consider the following: John received a call from a friend who was in significant distress over the loss of a loved one. John drove to his friend's house. On the way, he labored over what to say. When he arrived 30 minutes later, he was still unsure of what to say or do. Finally, John simply said to his friend, "I'm so sorry." For the next hour, John and his friend simply sat together in silence until John said, "What can I do for you?" His friend said, "Nothing . . . but thanks." John left feeling as though he had let his friend down. He didn't solve his problem. He didn't make his friend feel any better. Two days later John received a note from his friend. The note simply said, "Dear John, Thanks for all you did, I will never ever forget it." What did John do? He was present and his nonintrusive presence mattered.

Staying Calm — Equanimity

Presence is not enough. The type of presence matters. Demonstrating *equanimity*, or the ability to emit calmness and display self-confidence under pressure, can be an important aspect of an effective ministry of presence, especially in situations in which the person in distress feels out of control or fearful. Do not underestimate this skill; demonstrating calmness and confidence in the midst of an adverse situation sends a powerful, soothing message.

Communication Styles

To connect with someone initially, remember that human communication exists at two general levels: (1) cognitive (or thinking) and (2) emotional. In the absence of a critical incident, most people think first, or lead with their heads (i.e., cognitive), and then follow with their hearts (emotional). We all know people, however, who are the exception; they lead with their hearts or wear their emotions on their sleeve. However, in the aftermath of a critical incident, the usual dynamic of leading with one's head (cognition) sometimes shifts and results in people communicating more emotionally and thus less cognitively.

From the perspective of a PFA provider, gauge whether the person in the aftermath of a crisis situation is leading with his head or heart. Those leading cognitively typically seek information, whereas those leading emotionally usually seek more support. In the course of an encounter with someone who has experienced a critical incident, it is prudent, if possible, to try and implement a broad, overarching paradigm in which you help to (1) facilitate an initial cognitive perspective, (2) guide the person to a more emotional and personal perspective, and then (3) provide the individual with information to help her return to, or adapt to, a cognitive perspective.

Empathy and Rapport

To help facilitate cognitive or emotional communication styles, the constructs of empathy and rapport must be understood. Empathy is a genuine, nonjudgmental manner of responding in which the crisis interventionist is attuned to the range of meaning and emotions the person in crisis is experiencing and relates to them (Egan, 1994). It is considered the most important core feature in promoting a positive outcome when working with others (Orlando & Howard, 1986).

Empathy can be defined as *thinking as someone thinks and feeling as someone feels*. It is not sympathy. Sympathy may be thought of as *feeling for* someone. Sympathy can be helpful at times but implies expressing pity (Martin, 2011) and thus may undermine your efforts. Few people want to be felt sorry for. Empathy may be thought of as an advanced level of rapport, that is, connectedness.

The Empathic Cascade: The Bridge from Rapport to Adherence

Empathic cascade is a term we have chosen for the rather natural progression of connectedness with another human being. The steps in the empathic cascade are intuitive. Empathy denotes understanding. Understanding leads to trust. Trust fosters adherence. This cascade of human reactions will benefit you greatly, especially if you realize it results in willingness on the part of the other person to cooperate and follow your suggestions. Inclinations toward adherence are essential when motivating people to evacuate their homes, get a vaccination, not drink from natural water sources after a disaster, or not take their own lives. You also can see why rapport and empathy are essential aspects of hostage negotiations and suicide intervention. The development of rapport and empathy is essentially using verbal and nonverbal behavior to establish an atmosphere of safety, understanding, nonjudgmental acceptance, and respect that allows someone in need to accept interventions (Hill, 2009).

People are more willing to seek and accept help if they believe the person attempting to help them genuinely cares. Consider the following example shared by a police officer responding to a potential suicide call relayed to him by a 37-year-old female dispatcher. When the officer arrived at the scene and attempted to communicate with the 35-year-old man who had expressed to a 911 dispatcher his suicidal intent and plan to jump to his death off a building ledge, the suicidal individual did not want to speak with the police officer. Instead, the suicidal person insisted on speaking only with the dispatcher because she had apparently done a highly effective job establishing rapport by emitting empathy when initially speaking with him. The officer, recognizing the inherent power of rapport and the empathic cascade, facilitated direct communication between the suicidal man and the dispatcher rather than insisting on doing the talk-down intervention himself. The dispatcher was successful in getting the suicidal man to adhere to her suggestions to back away from the ledge and to allow the police officer to transport him to a hospital.

In a crisis situation, how you supportively attend to the person (your nonverbal responses), your ability to listen with intent, and your willingness and ability to observe how he reacts to the intervention serve as the cornerstones of effective crisis intervention. Before exploring the nonverbal and verbal behaviors that help foster successful PFA, establishing rapport often begins with an introduction of who you are and a statement of your purpose. For example, in a crisis situation, this might entail something like, "I'm Jim from the local disaster relief team. I'm here to listen and hopefully help you understand better the reactions you might be experiencing and to offer some suggestions that might help you better cope with this situation."

We will expand on the nonverbal and verbal behaviors that constitute reflective listening, but first some background.

Historical Development

A primary foundation of rapport building is conveying an attentive presence and a willingness to listen. Listening refers to the ability to capture and understand what is being communicated (Egan, 1994) and is the basis for effective psychological intervention. Consistent with the theme of this text, PFA is both an art and a science. There is an art to learning how to listen and effectively enter and understand someone else's world. There is a science to becoming acquainted with the factors and concepts involved in establishing a positive relationship with someone and using techniques to assist him. We will provide an overview of both of these constructs now.

Carl Rogers, a prominent twentieth-century psychologist who was a pioneer of the humanism movement of psychotherapy that emphasized the unique qualities of human freedom and personal growth, identified the following core conditions for successful counseling: empathic understanding (communicating caring and understanding), unconditional positive regard (acceptance of someone as a person of worth and value), and congruence (one's self-concept aligns with actual experience) (Rogers, 1957). Robert Carkhuff, who also believed that the relationship served as the basis for growth and development, expanded on Rogers's work to include conditions of respect (focusing on a person's positive attributes), immediacy (expressing what is transpiring in the here and now), confrontation (noting discrepancies between what someone says and what he or she is doing), concreteness (to focus and discuss relevant issues in specific terms), and self-disclosure (making one's self known to others) to account for effective counseling, and he developed listening skills to promote these effects (Carkhuff, 1969, 1971).

While these communication skills have served as the basis for therapy, they also have been adapted and used extremely effectively when responding to critical incidents. One of the most prominent examples of this adaptation has been in the development of hostage or crisis negotiation teams. Before the 1973 creation of the Hostage Negotiation Team (HNT) of the New York Police Department (NYPD)—the first unit created to deal specifically with crises and hostage situations—the standard police response to these emergency encounters entailed (1) demanding the person surrender immediately, and if he did not comply, then (2) police would lay siege to attempt to resolve the situation (Thompson, 2014). The NYPD HNT and subsequent HNTs have used alternative methods of conflict resolution predicated on basic communication skills and collaboration. More specifically, general communication skills and tactics in crisis and hostage negotiation situations include

- minimizing distractions;
- introducing oneself;
- ensuring safety;
- facilitating rapport by being respectful, direct, credible, and honest;
- being aware of one's volume, pace, and tone when speaking;
- adapting to the hostage takers' vocabulary;
- clarifying;
- information gathering; and
- problem solving (Miller, 2005).

These requisite skills are effective, and it's no coincidence that they form the foundational basis and mechanisms of action of PFA.

Mechanisms of Action

When responding to critical incidents, we are referring to people's *reactions* to a situation, not to the situation itself. Therefore, crisis interventionists providing PFA should focus on the person's perceptions and judgments of the incident and not necessarily on the event. To provide effective PFA, it is essential that you connect with the person as soon as possible. Crisis responders might have only minutes to cultivate an effective interpersonal relationship. Therefore, having the confidence and ability to form extremely rapid and trusting relationships are often considered the sine qua non of successful PFA. What makes this particularly challenging is that, unlike medical first-aid responders who typically have sophisticated equipment to assist them in their response, PFA providers must rely solely on their words, behaviors, and ability to listen to respond effectively. In other words, the crisis interventionist needs to use communication skills that involve active and reflective listening techniques to perceive nonverbal information, hear verbal information, and respond verbally and nonverbally to both types of information to establish rapport, empathy, and an effective, helping relationship. Following are the specific reflective listening skills that help to facilitate the initial stage, or the **R**, in the RAPID PFA model.

Nonverbal Behavior

The old saying "actions speak louder than words" actually has some empirical support. Nonverbal communication, such as body language (e.g., facial expressions, hand gestures, other body movements), and paralinguistics (tone or how the words are said, speech rate, etc.), which are also considered a form of nonverbal communication, have been demonstrated in a few laboratory studies to account for more than 90% of a conveyed message (Mehrabian, 1971). Although these data were not intended to apply to normal conversations (so it is challenging to place accurate quantitative relevance on typical verbal and nonverbal behavior), they do, however, suggest that body language and tone might be more accurate indicators of meaning and emotion than the words themselves. Therefore, in establishing and then in demonstrating general principles of listening, the PFA responder must pay attention to nonverbal behaviors, including how words are spoken. This attention applies to her nonverbal behaviors, as well as to what she observes in those receiving the intervention.

Nonverbal behavior sends a powerful message, and, more often than not, a first impression is based on appearance. Therefore, from the perspective of the crisis interventionist, emitting an overall sense of calmness and assurance is a valuable nonverbal behavior. As you respond to someone in the aftermath of a critical incident, nonverbal behaviors begin with attending to the person and awareness of your own behaviors, such as

- the grip of your handshake (is it firm),
- establishing and maintaining comfortable eye contact,
- sitting with an open and receptive posture (arms unfolded, legs uncrossed, and body leaning slightly forward),
- maintaining a comfortable interpersonal distance,
- being attentive (even if there are possible internal or outside distractions),
- being aware of facial expressions (e.g., nodding affirmatively, not frowning or yawning), and
- minimizing foot and leg movement.

However, be aware that there are optimal levels to most nonverbal behaviors. For example, too much eye contact might be perceived as staring, and too many head nods or excessive movement can be distracting.

When considering others' nonverbal behaviors, pay attention to their

- handshake (is it passive; is it cold and sweaty, indicating a sympathetic nervous system response; or is it extremely tight, indicating a lack of awareness or desperate efforts to control the situation);
- willingness and ability to maintain eye contact;
- evidence of the "thousand mile" stare, which is thought to be brought on by stressful events, causing one to block out his or her surroundings and stare off into nothing;
- facial expressions (e.g., blank, tearful, frowning);
- seating posture (e.g., slouched as if exasperated, arms folded suggesting defensiveness); and
- body movements (e.g., shaking legs suggesting anxiousness).

Be aware of cultural differences and norms when assisting others (see chapter 11). For example, some First Nation people and Aboriginal Australian groups consider sustained eye contact offensive and disrespectful, or they will avoid eye contact when talking about serious topics (Brammer & MacDonald, 1996; Ivey, 1994). Moreover, American and British people generally prefer more distance when communicating than do Hispanic and Middle Eastern people (Hill, 2009).

Paralinguistic Behaviors

Consider paralinguistic behaviors, such as silence and tone of voice. Silence can be a useful tool if it is used by the crisis interventionist to convey empathy and respect or to allow the person space and time to collect his thoughts and to talk uninterruptedly. Silence also conveys that the crisis interventionist is not trying to pressure the person into talking and has plenty of time to spend. However, beware: the person in need may perceive a crisis interventionist's excessive silence as distracting, as a sign of disinterest, or as an attempt to be challenging. Distrust may result, escalating the crisis situation. Therefore, while silence can be a useful tool, balance it. As with other nonverbal behaviors, the accepted use of silence varies by culture.

Regarding the paralinguistic variable of tone, the PFA provider must consider speaking slowly, clearly, and not too loudly. In addition, sometimes it is prudent for the PFA provider to complement his voice style with the style of the person he is trying to help. For example, speak softly and slowly if the person in need speaks that way, and speak faster if that's the person's speaking style. However, if the person's speech seems overly fast (i.e., pressured or manic), then it is better for the PFA provider to slow down his or her pacing to attempt to slow the other person down and to assess whether the individual is able to naturally adjust to a slower pace.

Closed-Ended and Open-Ended Questions

Open-ended and closed-ended questions are two broad types of questions one might ask, and from a PFA perspective, there is a rationale for when and why these different types of questions are used. Closed-ended questions ask for specific information and restrict the response options available. The most restrictive closed-ended questions are those that result in a yes or no response. Some common examples of closed-ended stems include *Do you, Don't you, Is this, Isn't this, Was it*. However, be careful; too many closed-ended questions in a row may be perceived as interrogative. Conversely, open-ended questions are exploratory and allow for the provision of more information. Stems for open-ended questions include *What, How, When, Where, Why*. Initially, work to limit the use of why questions. They are more difficult than closed-ended questions to answer and often make others feel judged and thus defensive. PFA providers should also be aware of using too many open-ended questions in succession because these questions can inadvertently convey lack of listening.

Understanding the benefits of both types of questions can be useful in crisis situations. Closed-ended questions might be used to try to help transition someone experiencing considerable initial affect and emotion to a more cognitive framework. Moreover, as noted in chapter 3, when people are stressed, they sometimes experience cortical inhibition, so they are not thinking clearly. Asking probing or initial open-ended questions might exacerbate this condition. Therefore, it is often prudent to begin with closed-ended questions, and then move to open-ended, exploratory questions.

PPFA providers should not ask question after question. Therefore, using reflective statements is advantageous in PFA interventions. Let's consider them now.

Reflective Listening Techniques

The primary goal of reflective listening is to make the other person feel understood. The most basic technique is to help those in distress to keep talking by using either nonlanguage words or simple, socially reinforcing or minimally encouraging words, such as *uh-huh, hmm, yeah, I see*, and *really*. These types of words positioned at the end of a person's statement or a pause in their statement can convey a sense of empathy as well as indicate that the PFA provider is giving up her turn to talk, encouraging the person in need to continue. Overuse of this simple tool, however, can be distracting.

Another type of reflective listening technique is *restatement*. Restatements repeat back to the person in distress the words she used. Restatements often contain fewer words than what the person said and attempt to highlight the relevance of what the person said in a concrete and clear way. They are often referred to as mirroring techniques because they reflect back to the person to help him hear what he is saying without interpretation or judgment. Restatements also provide a check for accurate listening and an opportunity for the person in need to pause and possibly be more introspective about what he is saying. This can be particular salient in a crisis situation in which emotions might be overwhelming and cortical inhibition might lead to confused thinking. Therefore, receiving accurate restatements allows the person in crisis to hear how his concerns sound to others. As with other techniques, overuse of restatement can be distracting.

One of the most commonly used and most powerful reflective techniques is the *summary paraphrase*. Basically, the purpose of the summary paraphrase is to capture and state (reflect) in your own words the important content of what someone has just said and to do so more concisely. A summary paraphrase might be inserted when the person in distress pauses while speaking or, most commonly, when he or she finishes speaking. It is intended to allow the person to continue speaking with only minimal interruption while communicating that she is being heard and understood. It also allows for clarification of content and promotes a verbal give-and-take. Stems for summary paraphrasing include *So, In other words, Sounds like,* or *What I'm hearing you say is.* It requires more sophistication than restatement because the PFA provider needs to be accurate in her summary. Although it allows for clarification of content and possibly a new perspective for the person in crisis to consider, it also is a closed-ended question. Therefore, someone experiencing severe cortical inhibition ("dumbing down") might respond to a summary paraphrase with a yes or a no response. If this occurs, it gives the PFA provider an indication of how severe the person's reactions and possible dysfunction might be.

Summary paraphrases can be used with cognitive content or emotional content. In the latter case, you would be paraphrasing the emotion expressed by the other person. A person's expression of emotion may come directly as she tells you specifically what emotions are being experienced, or the expression may come as indirect, nonverbal displays of emotion. Paraphrases of emotional content might sound like,

"You seem really upset."
"Perhaps you're feeling angry."
"You sound pretty depressed."
"You look pretty confident."
"Are you telling me you are really anxious right now?"

Paraphrasing is an effective tool to build empathy and rapport (it helps to demonstrate that the PFA provider is working hard to understand the person in distress), encourage cathartic ventilation, instill hope, and clarify expressions, avoiding costly misunderstanding. It also helps to validate emotions, which may defuse an emotional spiral, to regulate emotions, to reduce confusion, and to foster adherence. For those experiencing cortical inhibition, paraphrasing might enable the person in distress to better identify and accept his emotions. Awareness of cultural and even gender differences is important when reflecting emotions. People in the United States are generally encouraged to be open about their feelings, whereas people from some non-American cultures may be more reserved (Pedersen et al., 2002). Moreover, men, particularly in the United States, have historically not been as socialized as women to express their feelings (Cournoyer & Mahalik, 1995).

Action Directives

Action directives are helpful in providing someone in distress with concrete, specific answers if he asks a direct question or if specific courses of action are indicated. This can be helpful in a crisis, particularly if someone is evidencing cortical inhibition. It is usually best to provide a direct answer as long as that answer does not escalate the crisis. For example, if someone who works for a small, local company partially destroyed by a fire asks in the hours after the incident, "So I guess we're all going to lose our jobs?" it is probably better for the PFA responder to state, "I can understand your concern, but it seems worthwhile to wait for more information about the extent of the damage and what this means for the company" instead of "Looking at this damage, it's likely best for you and everyone else to start looking for new jobs."

Now that we have reviewed the basics of communication, including establishing rapport through nonverbal behavior, paralinguistic behavior, and active listening techniques, let us see how to apply these skills.

Demonstration of the R in RAPID Model

Understanding and establishing proficiency in the use of the RAPID model requires exposure and practice. We will explain each of the stages of the model in a separate chapter. However, to provide continuity and coherence, we will use the following pre-COVID-19 scenario, based on an amalgam of real situations, to provide a demonstration of dialogue that might occur between a PFA provider (crisis interventionist) and someone exposed to a traumatic event and expand it for each of the RAPID model stages. Let us start with the scenario and then demonstrate how rapport can be developed through nonverbal behaviors, paralinguistic behavior, and active listening techniques — the R in the RAPID model. Please note that unlike some of the other stages of the RAPID model, establishing rapport and using reflective listening techniques are invoked throughout the process.

Scenario

After two days of unusually heavy rain and unseasonable cold temperatures beginning on June 10 and culminating in a three-hour span on June 11 in which there were two to three inches of rain per hour, the South Platte River in Colorado crested nearly nine feet above its flood stage in some local areas. With very little warning, hundreds of homes in the surrounding counties were filled with as much as five feet of water and several roofs collapsed from the wind, rain, and falling trees causing almost total destruction of at least a dozen homes. Given the imminent needs of surrounding communities, it took up to 12 hours for emergency response units to respond to some of the residents and communities affected by the floods. More than 200 people were evacuated and sought shelter at local schools and houses of worship. By late morning of June 12, the bulk of the flooding had receded. However, the impact on roads, highways, bridges, and agricultural parcels was devastating. By 3 p.m. on June 12, most people were allowed to return to their homes. For some, it was returning to the remains of what used to be their homes.

In a preemptive effort to assist those returning to what is left of their homes, the local health department asks several individuals trained in PFA to be present and to assist those who might need assistance.

What follows is the initial contact with a flood survivor who also survived a tree that fell on her house. She stands in the mud-soaked street staring at the remains of what used to be her home. She appears to be in her late fifties or early sixties, she is motionless, and she's evidencing a thousand-mile stare while overlooking the rubble and debris in front of her. She appears particularly fixated on the 65-foot ponderosa pine tree that fell and crushed the roof of her house.

On the same side of the street, a man in his mid-forties, wearing a yellow windbreaker jacket, is standing and observing as people in the community return to assess the damage to their homes. He is trying to remain unassuming, but he can't help but be somewhat emotionally affected by what he is observing. After several minutes, he notices that the woman described previously is remaining motionless, with her eyes seemingly fixated on her yard littered with debris and the intimidating sight of the colossal tree that collapsed her roof and destroyed her house.

As he chooses to approach her, he notices that she does not initially appear to be in physical or medical distress. He stands next to her, establishing his presence, but she continues to stare ahead, apparently either oblivious to or ignoring him. He hesitates momentarily but then collects himself and decides to follow through with his objective. He is the crisis interventionist who will provide PFA.

MATT, *crisis interventionist*: Hello.

The woman remains silent (5 seconds).

MATT: I'm Matt from local disaster relief.

The woman remains silent (7 seconds).

MATT: I'm just checking . . . Are you able to hear me?

He looks at her and waits for a response. She continues to look straight ahead at the debris scattered across a yard and the enormous tree that has fallen.

WOMAN: This was mine.

MATT: This was your house?

Still looking straight ahead.

WOMAN: Yes.

MATT: Do you mind if I stand here with you?

WOMAN: No

Silence for 10 seconds.

MATT: Do you need anything?

WOMAN: Need anything? Like what?

MATT: Like something to drink or eat, or maybe a blanket?

WOMAN: I could use some water.

MATT: Are you okay if I leave you here for a moment? I have some water in my car.

WOMAN: That's fine.

MATT: Okay. Then let me get some water for you, and I'll be right back.

In about 90 seconds, Matt returns. As he approaches, she turns and acknowledges him.

MATT: Here's the water. Can I get you anything else?

WOMAN: No, thank you.

MATT: What should I call you?

She turns and extends her arm to shake his hand.

WOMAN: I'm Claire.

They shake hands; his grip is firm, hers is weak, and her palms are sweaty.

CLAIRE: And what did you say your name was?

MATT: I'm Matt from the local health department. I'd like to try and help you as best I can.

CLAIRE: What can you do to help me? It's all gone. I can't imagine I'll ever get through this.

MATT, *maintaining a sense of calmness and an evenness in the tone of his voice as he speaks:* I'm sorry. Events like this are incredibly hard to understand. But sometimes being able to talk about what happened, to understand better some of your reactions, and to talk about ways to help you get through it can be beneficial.

Silence (20 seconds).

CLAIRE: My husband, Jim, who died five years ago this month, worked in construction. We purchased what was little more than a shack 30 years ago and turned it into this beautiful home with a wraparound porch and a swing. *Pause.*

MATT: Hmm ... Thirty years ago, with a wraparound porch and a swing.

CLAIRE: Yeah. And the swing had a distinctive, rhythmic squeak that would happen only when we were both sitting and gliding on it. He was always looking for ways to make improvements to the house, and I would help whenever I could. Sometimes the best I could do was to make his favorite blueberry pie to enjoy when he was done working.

MATT: So this wasn't just a house, this was a *home* ... with sights, sounds, and smells that seemed to create some incredibly fond memories.

CLAIRE: Yeah, and now it's all gone ... along with Jim.

MATT: Sounds like some really tough losses.

CLAIRE: Jim was struggling with cancer for a number of years, so as sad as his death was when it occurred, in many ways it was a relief for me.

MATT: So, it seems that you didn't want Jim to suffer any longer than he had to?

CLAIRE: It was cruel to watch him suffer, but now our house is gone.

Silence (20 seconds).

And you know what makes it even worse?

MATT: Even worse?

CLAIRE: Look at the other houses around me. Sure, they have some water damage, but mine is gone. Gone! Why couldn't our house be the one that was spared! I mean, I'm a good person! Why? Why?

MATT: Claire, I can see that you're upset.

CLAIRE, *with tears forming in her eyes:* I'm sad and I'm hurt.

MATT: It just doesn't seem fair, does it?

Claire shakes her head in response.

CLAIRE: Not at all.

MATT: As I've said, I'll help you anyway I can. And if I can't help, I'll work to find resources that can help you. But one of the best ways for me to begin to help you is by listening to you tell me what happened. Are you okay to talk about it?

CLAIRE: Yeah.

Scenario Summary

Matt, the crisis interventionist, made contact with Claire after he perceived her as needing help, and he briefly introduced himself. He was present, and he emitted equanimity. He checked to make sure there were no physical or medical conditions occurring with her, including making sure she could hear him. This, we will see later, is consistent with the *assessment* phase of the RAPID model, which will be reviewed in more detail in chapter 6. Given her thousand-mile stare, it was likely prudent for him to use paralinguistic behaviors, such as silence and his even tone of voice, to help establish a rapport. At first he used closed-ended questions to gauge the possible extent of her cortical inhibition and to establish a preliminary cognitive framework from which to begin his questioning. Matt then used restatements, minimal encouragers, summary paraphrasing, and paraphrasing of emotion to help further establish rapport and empathy.

Because people often organize traumatic memories on a somato-sensory level (i.e., with their senses; van der Kolk, 1994), it was likely helpful for Matt to infuse aspects of how Claire was influenced by the sights, sounds, and smells of her home. He then continued to use these active listening skills as he gathered the beginning information of what transpired and her personal reactions to the critical incident. In particular, essential themes like belief in a safe and just world or fair-ness (which will be covered in detail in chapter 8), and the combined loss of her home and her husband are personal themes and reactions. Claire often used the phrase *our home* instead of *my home*, indicating the potential connection she maintains with her deceased husband. Matt has worked to establish rapport and has a developing sense of the type of person she is and what is important to her. He is now ready to inquire specifically about the event that occurred. This will happen during the assessment phase of the RAPID model, which will be cov-ered in chapter 6.

Mistakes to Avoid

In the aftermath of critical events, well-intentioned crisis interven-tionists may make common mistakes. They may not remain calm and probe too quickly for emotions and feelings without helping to reori-ent the person to a cognitive framework and then slowly transition-ing to inquiries about emotional aspects. Other common mistakes in-clude asking too many questions so that the person in crisis feels like she's being interrogated, rushing the person to answer questions, or making statements such as "I know how you feel," "It's not so bad," or "Others have it much worse." Using the same premise as the previous scenario, consider, for example, how the following exchange might not be effective:

MATT: Hello.

The woman remains silent (5 seconds).

MATT: I'm Matt from local disaster relief.

The woman remains silent (7 seconds).

This must be your house.

WOMAN: It was my house!

MATT: I'm so sorry. Wow! How are you feeling?

WOMAN: How am I feeling? Like my life has ended.

MATT: Your life hasn't ended. This is a setback, and you'll get through it. I know how you feel.

WOMAN: … having everything gone?

MATT: Losing material possessions can be sad, but they can be replaced. At least you're not injured physically. Are you? You seem to be experiencing more emotional pain. What's that like for you?

WOMAN: It feels awful!

MATT: I'm sorry, but it could have been worse.

WOMAN: Worse? How so?

MATT: Well, you fortunately were not in the house when the tree fell. And you have home insurance, don't you?

Asking the woman how she is feeling might lead her to experience a potential spiraling of emotions without establishing a sense of cognitive grounding. When the time seems appropriate to ask more emotional-type questions, our experience, at least with the emergency services culture, is to typically ask, "How are you doing with this?" compared to "How are you feeling about this?" to avoid the perception of being overly therapeutic or too touchy-feely. Also, in this current exchange, you can see where the crisis interventionist inserted statements about understanding how she is feeling and inadvertently trivialized her loss (he didn't ask, and therefore doesn't know, about the sentimental value attached to the home because of her husband). Moreover, the crisis interventionist did not use reflective statements and began asking irrelevant questions (i.e., about home insurance). Therefore, this exchange contained several instances of potentially ineffective ways to establish rapport and use reflective listening.

KEY POINT SUMMARY

1. Effective PFA is predicated on being present and communicating effectively.

2. People communicate on a cognitive and emotional level. Those who are more cognitively oriented are often seeking information, whereas those who are more affectively oriented are usually seeking support.

3. Listening is the foundation of communication, and this is evident in forms of psychotherapy. It has also been adapted by hostage and crisis negotiators when they respond to critical incidents.

4. Effective PFA is predicated on building rapport through equanimity (the ability to demonstrate calmness and confidence) and empathy (a genuine nonjudgmental manner of caring and responding).

5. Empathy represents understanding. Understanding leads to trust, which, in turn, leads to adherence. This is what we refer to as the *empathic cascade*.

6. The PFA provider should be aware of how nonverbal behavior (e.g., facial expressions, body movements) and paralinguistics (tone, rate of speech, use of silence) affect rapport.

7. Be aware of how verbal behavior (open-ended and close-ended questions) and active listening techniques (restatement, summary paraphrasing, paraphrasing of emotion, and action directives) impact rapport and empathy.

8. The effective (and ineffective) use of rapport established through active listening was illustrated using a disaster scenario, which will be built upon in the next four chapters as well to demonstrate how to employ the remaining parts of the RAPID PFA model.

References

Brammer, L. M., & MacDonald, G. (1996). *The helping relationship: Process and skills* (6th ed.). Boston, MA: Allyn & Bacon.

Carkhuff, R. R. (1969). *Helping and human relations* (Vols. 1–2). New York, NY: Holt, Rinehart, & Winston.

Carkhuff, R. R. (1971). *The development of human resources: Education, psychology, and social change.* New York, NY: Holt, Rinehart, & Winston.

Cournoyer, R. J., & Mahalik, J. R. (1995). Cross-sectional study of gender role conflict examining college-aged and middle-aged men. *Journal of Counseling Psychology, 19*, 11–19. http://dx.doi.org/10.1037/0022-0167.42.1.11.

Egan, G. (1994). *The skilled helper: A model for systematic helping and interpersonal relating* (5th ed.). Monterey, CA: Brooks/Cole.

Hill, C. E. (2009). *Helping skills: Facilitating exploration, insight, and action* (3rd ed.). Washington, DC: American Psychological Association.

Ivey, A. E. (1994). *Intentional interviewing and counseling: Facilitating client development in a multicultural society* (3rd ed.). Pacific Grove, CA: Brooks/Cole.

Martin, D. (2011). *Counseling and therapy skills* (3rd ed.). Long Grove, IL: Waveland Press.

Mehrabian, A. (1971). *Silent messages.* Oxford, UK: Wadsworth.

Miller, L. (2005). Hostage negotiation: Psychological principles and practice. *International Journal of Emergency Mental Health, 7*, 277–298.

Orlando, D. E., & Howard, K. I. (1986). Process and outcome in psychotherapy. In S. L. Garfield & A. E. Bergin (Eds.), *Handbook of psychotherapy and behavior change* (pp. 431–441). New York, NY: Wiley.

Pedersen, P. B., Draguns, J. G., Lonner, W. J., & Trimble, J. E. (2002). *Counseling across cultures* (5th ed.). Thousand Oaks, CA: Sage.

Rogers, C. R. (1957). The necessary and sufficient conditions of therapeutic personality change. *Journal of Counseling Psychology, 21*, 95–103. http://dx.doi .org/10.1037/h0045357.

Thompson, J. (2014, March 5). "Crisis" or "hostage" negotiation? The distinction between two important terms. *FBI Law Enforcement Bulletin.* https://leb.fbi.gov/2014/march/crisis-or-hostage-negotiation-the -distinction-between-two-important-terms.

Thorne, F. C. (1952). Psychological first aid. *Journal of Clinical Psychology, 8*, 210–211.

van der Kolk, B. (1994). The body keeps score: Memory and the evolving psychobiology of posttraumatic stress. *Harvard Review of Psychiatry, 1*, 253–265. http://dx.doi.org/10.3109/10673229409017088.

six | **A**—Assessment

Listening to the Story

AFTER ESTABLISHING CONTACT and rapport with a person in distress, the Johns Hopkins RAPID PFA model progresses to the *assessment* of basic physical and psychological needs. The essential criterion searched for, and focused on, is evidence of impairment or dysfunction. This rudimentary evaluation does not rely on structured psychometric assessment (e.g., objective questionnaires or a structured interview); rather, it is derived from a guided conversation involving the survivor's personal narrative. It is sometimes thought of as the survivor's *story* or as the *context* for intervention. This evaluative conversation is punctuated with specific questions posed by the interventionist to direct the flow of the conversation and to clarify specific aspects of the story. Remember that the *intervention* phase is largely predicated on the idiosyncratic needs of the person in distress. These needs will be revealed to you in the assessment phase as the person in distress describes the personal reactions experienced in the wake of some event (critical incident) as well as a brief description of the situational context for the reactions (i.e., the incident itself). Thus, to formulate your intervention, you must listen carefully and nonjudgmentally to the story.

Remember, the story consists of two elements: (1) a rudimentary disclosure of the critical event (i.e., what happened) and (2) the person's reactions to the event. The story is not complete until you have some information pertaining to both elements.

Assessment is ideally unobtrusive and typically brief in most acute contexts. It is also a consensus core psychological first aid (PFA) competency identified in the seminal McCabe et al. (2014) report. Assessment encompasses two dynamic processes: (1) screening and (2) appraisal. These evaluative processes are designed to differentiate functionally discrete subsamples of PFA recipients according to magnitude of need for PFA intervention. It is comparable to determining the need to stop arterial bleeding in physical first aid.

Screening

The first step in assessment entails screening. Screening consists of an attempt to answer prefatory, or qualifying, binary (yes-no) questions; for example, three key questions should be considered:

1. Is there any evidence that this person needs assistance?
2. Is there any evidence that this person's ability to adaptively function and attend to her necessary responsibilities is being, or may be, compromised?
3. Is further exploration into this person's capacity for adaptive mental and behavioral functioning warranted?

To assist in answering these three questions, you may draw inferences from the following domains:

1. Integrity of physical health
2. Physical safety
3. Psychophysiological distress
4. Cognitive and intellectual functioning
5. Affective and behavioral expression
6. Interpersonal resources
7. Material resources

Differentiating functional and dysfunctional behavior rests on a general understanding of the human stress response as discussed in chapter 3 (Cannon, 1932; Everly & Lating, 2019; Selye, 1956) and familiarity with activities of daily living and the person-specific instrumental activities associated with daily living (Katz et al., 1970; Lawton & Brody, 1969). These are important constructs borrowed from psychiatric recovery and rehabilitation contexts that refer to the ability to maintain everyday activities associated with personal hygiene, homemaking, employment, financial management, childcare, and eldercare.

If the answer is "no," to each of the three questions posed above, then no further attention is likely warranted at that time. However, this does not preclude a subsequent follow-up. If, the answer is "yes" to any of the three questions, then further inquiry is warranted. To do so, you would move to appraisal.

Appraisal

If the screening process indicates that additional inquiry is warranted, then you transition from binary screening to dimensional appraisal. Appraisal poses dimensional questions, for example:

> To what extent is there any evidence that this person needs assistance?; or

> To what extent is there any evidence that this person's ability to adaptively function and attend to his necessary responsibilities is being, or may be, compromised?

Lists of potential signs, or indicia, of *distress* (significant but sub-impairment stress arousal) and *dysfunction* (impaired stress arousal) follow. They are not comprehensive but, rather, list potential examples. They are divided into cognitive, emotional, behavioral, spiritual, and physiological indicia. Evidence indicates that some disturbance in activities of daily living is more the rule than the exception in the wake of significant critical incidents, especially disasters (see Everly & Parker, 2005, for a review). Nevertheless, most people in the aftermath of a critical incident appear resilient without any assistance (Bonnano, 2004). Therefore, the dimensional assessment of the extent of dysfunction is critical to avoiding (1) wasting resources on unnecessary interventions and (2) interfering with the natural trajectory of one's personal resilience.

Cognitive Indicia

Distress

- Temporary confusion, time distortion, dyscalculia (difficulty doing math)
- Inability to concentrate
- Reduced problem-solving capacity
- Feeling overwhelmed, overloaded
- Obsessions
- Reliving the event
- Nightmares

Dysfunction

- Incapacitating confusion, diminished cognitive capacity
- Hopelessness
- Suicidal thoughts
- Homicidal thoughts
- Hallucinations
- Paranoid delusions
- Inability to prioritize important tasks
- Evidence of dissociation (rule out acute psychosis)

Emotional Indicia

Distress

- Fear
- Sadness
- Irritability
- Anger

- Frustration
- Bereavement–loss
- Anxiety

Dysfunction

- Panic attacks
- Immobilizing depression
- Affective/emotional numbing
- Acute or posttraumatic stress disorder

Behavioral Indicia
Distress

- Temporary phobic avoidance
- Compulsions
- Hoarding
- Sleep disturbance
- Eating disturbance
- Easily startled
- Reticence (being reserved)

Dysfunction

- Persistent avoidance
- Immobilizing compulsions
- Aggression–violence
- Reclusiveness
- Impulsiveness, risk taking
- Self-medication
- Alcohol abuse
- Abusing prescription drugs
- Abusing energy drinks
- Inability to speak or respond to cues
- Catatonia (abnormality of movement or behavior)

Spiritual Indicia

Distress

- Questioning faith
- Questioning God's actions

Dysfunction

- Cessation of faith-related practices
- Projecting faith onto others

Physiological Indicia

Distress

- Disturbance in appetite
- Disturbance in libido
- Psychogenic headaches
- Psychogenic muscle aches/spasms
- Decreased immunity (increased colds, infections last longer)

Note: Any prolonged physical/physiological changes or any symptoms of concern should be evaluated by a medical professional.

Dysfunction

- Changes in cardiac function
- Changes in gastrointestinal function
- Detection of occult blood (blood in the stool not visible to the naked eye)
- Unconsciousness
- Chest pain
- Dizziness
- Numbness/paralysis (especially of arm, leg, face)

Note: Seek medical care for all of these symptoms.

Demonstration of the A in RAPID Model

Let us return to the scenario and see how the tools of assessment can be highlighted in the RAPID model. Again, recall that reflective listening techniques will be implemented throughout the RAPID process, so note how these are used as Claire tells her story of what occurred, and Matt screens and then appraises her functioning.

MATT, *crisis interventionist*: So, what happened?

CLAIRE: The rain started two days ago, and it just wouldn't stop. After the first day, I was worried about my basement flooding, so I kept checking my sump pump, but it seemed to be doing okay.

MATT: Um hmm. So, you were concerned and kept checking the sump pump?

CLAIRE: Yes, it takes a lot of rain for flooding to occur in the basement, but by the second day, I was becoming more and more concerned. The news reports kept talking about flash floods and roads becoming impassable.

MATT: Did you need to go anywhere?

CLAIRE: No, thank goodness. I was able to stay home.

MATT: Okay. That was good for you.

CLAIRE: It was good for me at the time, but by the evening of the second day of the storm, when it really started coming down, the entire neighborhood lost power, and my basement started flooding very rapidly. Jim always wanted to install a backup generator, but he never quite got around to it.

MATT: So it's pouring rain, you lose power, you're alone, and water is now rushing into your basement. This was all probably getting pretty scary?

CLAIRE: To say the least. I wasn't sure what to do and I was having a difficult time thinking straight.

MATT: When you say you weren't thinking straight, what do you mean?

CLAIRE: I started feeling like I had to do things very quickly and that my mind was racing a bit. I started to move things out of the basement, but I wasn't sure at the time what was most important. I wish I would have grabbed the photo albums.

MATT: So your mind is racing a bit, and you wished you had grabbed the photo albums?

CLAIRE: Yes, of Jim and our daughter, Marissa. She lives in Arizona now with her husband who's an attorney, and my three-year-old granddaughter, Caitlin. Marissa was in constant contact with me during the storm and encouraged me to get out of the house once the water in the basement started rising.

MATT: So what did you do?

CLAIRE: Before I knew what to do, my next-door neighbor, one of the ones whose house is relatively undamaged, called me because she was worried that I was alone. She insisted that I come over and stay with her and her husband. So I grabbed what I could carry and went to their house. I was convinced that nothing more than a little water in the basement was going to happen though . . .

MATT: You didn't want to think, let alone believe, something worse could happen.

CLAIRE: . . . but I was wrong.

Silence for 15 seconds.

When I arrived at my neighbors' house, they had candles lit, and we sat and talked about what we could do, and then we heard on their battery-operated radio that a shelter was being set up within the hour at the local parish located on top of a hill less than a mile away. While sitting there with them, I noticed that my hands were cold, clammy, and shaky, and my mouth was very dry. I asked for something to drink and the water seemed to help. As we were in the house preparing to leave for the shelter, we heard what sounded like waves of water, and then the sound of wood snapping. We ran to the window and I watched in disbelief, almost horror, as an enormous pine tree came crashing down on our house . . . it was completely crushed. It was the worst thing I've ever seen. If this wasn't bad enough, I then watched as the water started carrying away large parts of our home . . . the roof, the porch, the swing. I was speechless, and I shut down. I wanted to simply sit and cry, but I couldn't move.

Claire now looking at the rubble.

MATT: What an awful experience for you. The power of nature is amazing and humbling. It can often leave us feeling out of control.

CLAIRE: Yeah. That's for sure.

MATT: It seems that what you wanted to do was stop, absorb, and process all that was happening, including some of your physical reactions, but it doesn't sound like that's what you were able to do?

CLAIRE: No. I had to keep moving because we decided to go to the shelter.

MATT: What was that like?

CLAIRE: Since it was so close, we were able to get there with little difficulty. My neighbor's husband drove. When we arrived, there were about 30 other people there, most of whom I know from the community, and we heard from them how difficult some of the roads were. Although it was nice to be around others and feel their support, I really wanted to be left alone. I couldn't stop thinking about what happened to our house.... I just kept seeing the tree fall over and over again ... it was like it was happening in slow motion. I felt numb.

MATT: So while you appreciated the support of others, you wanted to be left alone, and it sounds like you couldn't stop thinking about the tree falling?

CLAIRE: It just didn't seem real. I wanted ... no, I needed, to get back here as soon as possible so I could see it again ... and this is where you found me.

MATT: Our minds try to protect us, so sometimes it's hard to initially believe that something like this is actually true.

Claire, staring at the debris and the tree.

CLAIRE: I'm looking right at it now, and I'm still having a hard time believing it's true. I'm feeling really helpless right now.

MATT: I'm sorry. This must be really tough.

CLAIRE: . . . it sure is, but in this instance, seeing is unfortunately believing.

MATT: Claire, I want to make sure I'm hearing what you're saying and what's important to you. You just mentioned feeling helpless. And earlier you noted that before you went to your neighbors' home, you had some difficulty thinking clearly. You then mentioned that your hands were cold, clammy, and shaky, and that your mouth was dry when you were at your neighbors'. When you went to the shelter, you said you wanted to be left alone. Are there other signs of distress you have experienced?

CLAIRE: Like what?

MATT: Well, sometimes people in the aftermath of situations like this have a difficult time eating or sleeping.

CLAIRE: Well, when I went to the shelter, they had some food there, but I just wasn't hungry, so I didn't eat. They also had cots set up for us to sleep on, but I had a very difficult time getting to sleep that night. In fact, when I did fall asleep, I had nightmares about trees falling. When I woke up this morning, I felt like a combination of shock mixed with anger. I was hoping that once I came back here, I'd feel less depressed.

MATT: Given what you've been through, what you're describing is not unusual at all, and I want to talk more about that in a bit. However, before we do, I wanted to first ask you about what you mean when you say you're feeling depressed. What does depression feel like for you?

CLAIRE: Hmm . . . sad . . . empty, and lonely, I guess. But I imagine that feelings of depression after losing everything you own are likely pretty common. I'm sure there are a lot of people around here feeling the same.

MATT: You're probably right . . . but it's important to remember that everyone is different.

Have you had any other physical reactions?

CLAIRE: I'm feeling an odd combination of fatigue and restlessness. And now I'm waking up today realizing that I'm homeless.

Scenario Summary

Matt was able to use the rapport he had built, along with reflective listening, to allow his assessment, in other words, screening and appraisal, to occur while Claire was telling her story. In regards to the three key binary questions noted at the beginning of the chapter regarding screening, Claire certainly seems to need assistance. Her ability to function adaptively seems somewhat compromised, and further exploration of her capacity for adaptive functioning seems warranted. Claire shows evidence of psychophysiological distress and affective dysfunction and has lost some of her most valued material possessions. Moreover, in working to appraise the extent of her need for assistance, along with gauging her level of adaptive functioning, it is notable that she is reporting nightmares, some diminished capacity to concentrate, fear, avoidance, diminished appetite, sadness, and loss. Matt has done a good job collecting these pieces of information and paraphrasing them back to Claire. Most of the extent of the signs and symptoms Claire is currently reporting are consistent with distress, as compared to more extreme indicators of dysfunction. For example, she seems to able to take care of her daily living needs, although there is some concern about her lack of appetite. Matt will need to focus initially on his appraisal of the circumstances and symptoms that he believes are more important and impact Claire most saliently. This *prioritization* will be covered in the next chapter.

Mistakes to Avoid

Claire provided clear examples of emotional (e.g., fear, sadness, loss) and behavioral (e.g., cold clammy hands, dry mouth, avoidance, sleep disturbance) distress. A beginner PFA provider may want to fix the problems a person in distress describes, often by normalizing her reported reactions as soon as they are expressed. Resist this urge to intervene early in the assessment process. As you will see, there will be time and more suitable opportunity during the *intervention* stage to provide explanatory and anticipatory guidance (see chapter 8). For example, consider the following exchange between Claire and Matt wherein he inappropriately rushes to provide explanations:

CLAIRE: While sitting there with them, I noticed that my hands were cold, clam——

MATT, *interrupting before she can finish:* Having cold hands is a normal reaction. It's part of your how your sympathetic nervous system responds . . . blood, which is warm, does not flow as freely to your extremities when you're nervous.

CLAIRE: I also was going to say that my hands were clammy, and that . . .

MATT, *again interrupting:* I want you to know that's normal, too. Your hands breaking out in a cold sweat is part of the nervous system response.

CLAIRE: . . . and my mouth was dry.

MATT: Also normal, Claire. Your digestive system has shut itself down, and since saliva is the first part of digestion, your mouth becomes dry. So can you see how all of these responses are normal?

While the information Matt is sharing with Claire is accurate, and even though he is well intentioned, the timing and the repetitive, if not intrusive, nature of his responses have the potential to overwhelm Claire and to inhibit the progression of *her* story or her willingness to tell it. This results in limited ability to assess fully how she is presenting.

Another possible mistake, and one that will be addressed in more depth in the intervention chapter, is misinterpreting or overpathologizing what someone says. In this scenario, when Claire said that she was feeling depressed, Matt subtly normalized the reaction, but then asked for clarification from Claire about what depression means to her. Consider, instead, the following exchange:

CLAIRE: I was hoping that once I came back here, I'd feel less depressed.

MATT: So you're aware of what it's like to be depressed? Have you
been treated for depression? Depression is sometimes related to
suicidal thoughts so we can't be too careful.

Matt's response in this situation is abrupt and possibly overpathologizing Claire's presentation. He then seems to infer that Claire may
be suicidal, which could be traumatizing to her. If there was any hint
of suicidal thinking, Matt certainly should have inquired further, but
to go there prematurely, simply on the basis of her use of the term *depression*, is problematic. When people use ambiguous terms, such as
anxiety, *depression*, and *panic*, be sure to clarify what they mean before
jumping to conclusions.

KEY POINT SUMMARY

1. Although seemingly redundant, assessment consists of two dynamic processes: screening and appraisal.
2. Screening consists of posing to yourself three binary questions:
    a. Is there any evidence that this person needs assistance?
    b. Is there any evidence that this person's ability to adaptively
       function and attend to her necessary responsibilities is be-
       ing, or may be, compromised?
    c. Is further exploration into this person's capacity for adap-
       tive mental and behavioral functioning warranted?
3. On the basis of an affirmative response to any of the three questions, you then progress to appraisal.
4. Appraisal is a dimensional process wherein the following questions
   are asked:
    a. *To what extent* is there any evidence that this person needs
       assistance?
    b. *To what extent* is there any evidence that this person's abil-
       ity to adaptively function and attend to her necessary re-
       sponsibilities is being, or may be, compromised?
5. Assessment is a precursor to psychological triage.
6. The figure included here summarizes the steps in the assessment
   phase of the RAPID model.

Figure 6.1   Steps of *assessment* in RAPID PFA

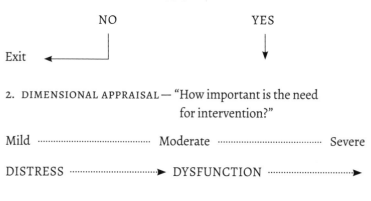

1. BINARY SCREENING — "Is there any evidence of need for PFA/psychosocial intervention?"

NO   YES

Exit

2. DIMENSIONAL APPRAISAL — "How important is the need for intervention?"

Mild ·· Moderate ································ Severe

DISTRESS ································▶ DYSFUNCTION ·······························▶

References

Bonnano, G. A. (2004). Loss, trauma, and human resilience: Have we underestimated the human capacity to thrive after extremely aversive events? *American Psychologist, 59,* 20–28. http://dx.doi.org/10.1037/0003-066X.59.1.20.

Cannon, W. B. (1932). *The wisdom of the body.* New York, NY: Norton.

Everly, G. S., Jr., & Lating, J. M. (2019). *A clinical guide to the treatment of the human stress response* (4th ed.). New York, NY: Springer Nature.

Everly, G. S., Jr., & Parker, C. L. (Eds.). (2005). *Mental health aspects of disaster: Public health preparedness and response.* Baltimore, MD: Johns Hopkins Center for Public Health Preparedness.

Katz, S., Downs, T. D., Cash, H. R., & Grotz, R. C. (1970). Progress in development of the index of ADL. *Gerontologist, 10,* 20–30. http://dx.doi.org/10.1093/geront/10.1_Part_1.20.

Lawton, M. P., & Brody, E. M. (1969). Assessment of older people: Self-maintaining and instrumental activities of daily living. *Gerontologist, 9,* 179–186. http://dx.doi.org/10.1093/geront/9.3_Part_1.179.

McCabe, O. L., Everly, G. S., Jr., Brown, L. M., Wendelboe, A. M., Abd
Hamid, N. H., Tallchief, V. L., & Links, J. M. (2014). Psychological first aid:
A consensus-derived, empirically supported, competency-based training
model. *American Journal of Public Health, 104,* 621–628. http://dx.doi.org
/10.2105/AJPH.2013.301219.

Selye, H. (1956). *The stress of life.* New York, NY: McGraw-Hill.

SEVEN | P—Psychological Triage

Prioritization

PSYCHOLOGICAL TRIAGE is the designation of relative urgency. The term *triage* has a French derivation that means to create a hierarchy for selection. In medical terms, triage means a sorting of survivors or patients by order of urgency for care. More specifically, psychological triage refers to a process by which you prioritize attendance to people according to their relative urgency of need for psychological first aid (PFA) and psychosocial support.

In the previous chapter, we discussed the steps in assessment. We said global assessment consisted of two constituent dynamic processes: (1) the binary process of screening (the search for evidence of need for intervention) and (2) the more dimensional process of the appraisal of the importance, or gravity, of need. Thus, assessment is the determination of the *presence and importance of need* for PFA and other forms of intervention. Psychological triage, however, is a determination of the order in which the interventionist attends to (1) recipients (when there are more than current resources can attend to); (2) their respective signs and symptoms; and most important, (3) their specific needs. It is in effect the creation of a hierarchy of *relative urgency.* Psychological triage is not a mutually exclusive stage in RAPID, rather it is best understood as a seamless continuation of the overall assessment process in PFA that began with screening. The consensus report on PFA by McCabe et al. (2014) lists preintervention triage as a core competency preceding specific PFA intervention (which will be addressed in the chapter 8). So let's take a closer look at psychological triage.

Urgency

What determines urgency of need for PFA or psychosocial intervention? In emergency medicine, triage urgency is determined by the demand for survivability. More specifically, triage refers to a qualitative selection process based on the severity of a wound or illness, coupled with the overall suitability for treatment or intervention. In PFA, psychological triage is more complicated. Survivability is certainly a key determining factor, but there are other considerations.

Abraham Maslow (1970) developed a hierarchy for human motivation that serves as a useful beginning framework for determining relative degrees of urgency. Maslow considered physical and safety needs as the most fundamental. We would offer a more specific perspective by noting that medical/physiological (medical stability, water, food) needs should be first. Physical safety and meeting other physical needs (e.g., shelter) would also be primary.

After these more basic Maslovian needs are met, you should consider behavioral/psychosocial needs. The most important of all the behavioral/psychosocial needs is the ability to attend to one's daily responsibilities (e.g., childcare, eldercare, employment, self-care/hygiene, reconstruction or moving forward at the appropriate time). Significant impairment or dysfunction within these responsibilities can have serious and ripple-like effects, adversely affecting other individuals and delaying the overall course of reconstruction and recovery.

Thus, triage proficiency assumes knowledge of behavioral, or response-based, criteria for identifying impairments to essential activities of daily living, less important instrumental activities of daily living, and key empirically based predictors of subsequent posttraumatic illness and dysfunction. Indeed, certain aspects of the survivor's experience are considered predictors of posttraumatic disorders, and you should be careful to listen for those as well as issues that involve activities of daily living. Generally accepted, empirically based predictors of posttraumatic illness and dysfunction include, but are not limited to, the following:

1. Severity (intensity multiplied by duration of trauma exposure)
2. Post-event-perceived guilt; negative appraisal of self
3. Peritraumatic dissociation (occurring around the time of the trauma)
4. Peritraumatic depression (occurring around the time of the trauma)
5. Perceived life threat
6. Prior psychiatric history, especially acute stress disorder or posttraumatic stress disorder
7. Lack of perceived social support
8. Seeing human remains
9. Head injury (concussion, traumatic brain injury) (see Brewin, Andrews, & Valentine, 2000; Everly, 1999; Kleim, Ehlers, & Glucksman, 2007; and Ozer et al., 2003, for reviews and meta-analyses).

The presence of any or all of these factors can be revealed and prioritized by simply talking with the person (or other reliable sources of these data) and integrating his or her responses with your objective appraisal of the situation.

Psychological or Behavioral Instability: The Crisis Triad

So far we have given you the critical factors you should listen for and observe during triage. We have not overwhelmed you at this juncture with the criteria surrounding specific psychiatric diagnostic categories provided as an overview in chapter 3. However, there may be value in mentioning specific patterns of reactions that might serve to interfere with daily living and one's ability to move on to reconstruction and closure after a traumatic incident. There appear to be three recurrent constellational themes of *psychological/behavioral instability*. These three co-varying constellations may be referred to as the *crisis triad* and consist of the following:

1. Tendencies for behavioral impulsivity
2. Diminished cognitive capabilities (insight, recall, problem solving), but most important a diminished ability to understand the consequences of one's actions
3. An acute loss of future orientation or a feeling of helplessness.

The crisis triad is not only common but may be a latent syndrome in the majority of clinical psychiatric syndromes observed in the wake of adversity (Everly & Mitchell, 1999). Most important they serve to interfere with one's ability to attend to daily responsibilities.

Putting It All Together: The A-B-C Model of Psychological Triage

Alan Lakein (1973) authored an influential book on time management in the early 1970s that applies in the current discussion of psychological services following disasters and other critical incidents. Lakein argued that the preservation of resources is essential and that time is an essential resource. This is certainly true for the public health response to critical incidents such as Hurricane Katrina, tsunamis in Asia, and terrorist attacks in Paris. We know that the mental health surge will usually exceed the mental health surge capacity unless we use new models of service provision (Everly & Parker, 2005). We know that the longer we wait to intervene for posttrauma syndromes the more difficult mitigation and treatment become. Therefore, intervention resources and time are precious commodities. This is the whole premise behind PFA and the importance of effective assessment and triage.

Lakein noted that the demands on our time come in three categories: A, B, and C.

A = Important and urgent
B = Important not urgent, or urgent not important
C = Neither important nor urgent

Lakein suggests that we attend only to the As in our lives. The mistake that most people make is to attend to Bs. He says that Bs are demands in transition. Most Bs become Cs. Those Bs that become As then warrant attention. To attend to all Bs is to waste time and resources on demands that will take care of themselves.

We argue that the mental and behavioral consequences of disaster and adversity correspond accordingly to these three domains. You will encounter people with the following needs:

A— People who are highly impaired, dysfunctional, and suffering psychologically or physically. They are mostly in need of PFA and perhaps other types of support.

B— People who are resilient in the wake of adversity. They experience increased distress, even possible acute dysfunction that resolves with respite and informal support. Most survivors will be in this category.

C— People who are resistant to adversity. They are functional, if not often heroic.

From the PFA perspective, you should directly attend to As, monitor Bs, and leave Cs alone. In situations that are not acutely life threatening, the passage of time is usually helpful in de-escalating a volatile situation and in eroding symptoms of distress. This is an important lesson for crisis interventionists, therapists, and public health planners to learn.

Demonstration of the **P** in RAPID Model

Now that the assessment process has started, Matt must prioritize the relevant *urgency* of what Claire has said. Matt began this process early on in his exchange with Claire. For example, he ruled out that she was physically injured. In addition, even though she showed signs of distress, as detailed in chapter 6, he determined that she was lucid and able to communicate. In accordance with the crisis triad, Claire is currently not demonstrating or expressing tendencies for behavioral impulsivity, a diminished ability to understand the consequences of her actions, or an acute loss of future orientation. Matt should, however, pay attention to the possible intensity of her exposure based on her account of witnessing the tree destroying her house. Let's pick up their exchange.

MATT, *crisis interventionist*: I'm sorry your home is gone. I guess that is the literal definition of being homeless. Have you been able to consider where you will be staying?

CLAIRE: Well, the church offered me the opportunity to stay there as long as I'd like. That's very kind of them. My daughter, Marissa, also has offered to have me come to Arizona to stay with her, her husband, and my granddaughter. That sounds like a good idea maybe in the next couple of weeks but not right now.

MATT: Not right now?

CLAIRE: I really feel that there are things I need to take care of with the house before I travel there. But last night while I was at the church, I called my sister who lives about 20 minutes away, primarily to check on her.

MATT: That is very thoughtful. And how is she doing?

CLAIRE: Her home was not impacted that badly ... only a couple of inches of water in the basement. Like me, she lives by herself. When I told her what happened to my house, she became tearful. She knows what this house meant to me ... and Jim.

MATT: It sounds like your sister is very caring?

CLAIRE: She's three years older and has always been my protector ... [*seven-second pause*] ... my guardian angel.

MATT: Seems like a good time to have a guardian angel.

CLAIRE, *half smiling*: You're right! She asked ... well, more like insisted, that I'd come stay with her as long as I want. She said she'll enjoy the company. I just know that for the next couple of days I'll want to return here to see what personal things I can salvage. Who knows, maybe I'll find some of the photo albums.

MATT: So it sounds like you have a place to stay that is safe. And that being with your sister will provide you with support and comfort. That's very important, Claire.

CLAIRE: I feel fortunate that I have options. Do you know what else I feel fortunate, if not better, about?

MATT: Better about . . . what's that?

CLAIRE: I ate well this morning. They had oatmeal and fruit at the church, and I feel slightly embarrassed to admit it, but I ate two bowls.

MATT: Two bowls. Good for you. Have you eaten since?

CLAIRE: I typically don't eat lunch and usually eat dinner early, so I feel like I'll be hungry in the next couple of hours.

MATT: That's good. Your body is looking for food as its source of energy.

CLAIRE: Yeah, I have some work to do. I need to muster the energy to go through the remains of my house.

MATT: What's that going to be like for you . . . going through your house?

CLAIRE: I know I need to do it, but it's hard to get the image and sound of the tree falling out of my mind. It's like I'm afraid that something else, even another tree, might fall on me while I'm sorting through our belongings.

MATT: How real does that feel for you?

CLAIRE: I realize that it's highly unlikely given that the storm is over, but the intensity of the crash seems to be sticking with me . . . making me jumpy.

MATT: It was certainly an intense event, and your reactions are understandable.

CLAIRE: . . . but I'm not going to let them keep me from doing what I need to do.

Scenario Summary

Matt again used reflective statements to help foster rapport. From a Maslovian hierarchy of needs perspective, as well as determining what is urgent or important, it was prudent for Matt to focus on her basic physiological needs. In particular, making sure she had a place to stay and determining that she's eating. Claire also revealed to Matt that the intensity of the event was resonating with her and that she had some trepidation about sorting through the debris. Her reservation did not reach the level of dysfunction, but it is important to her and likely warrants ongoing appraisal. However, it was encouraging that, despite all that was occurring with her, Claire appeared to have energy and even a sense of recognition that things could be worse. Given the conversation with Claire revealed no urgent demands that warranted immediate attention, all of this information will now set the stage for and guide intervention.

Potential Mistakes to Avoid

During the RAPID process, sometimes providers fail to consider or forget to address prioritization. Moreover, sometimes PFA providers encourage people to focus on spending time with others (affiliation) and feeling better about themselves before establishing whether their basic physiological needs—for shelter, food, and water—have been met. Try not to let the following exchange occur:

MATT: I'm sorry your home is gone. But I'm glad you weren't hurt.

CLAIRE: Yes, I guess I should be thankful about that.

MATT: And . . . you did the best you could to not only get out of the house before the tree fell, but to go to a place where you could be around other people.

CLAIRE: Yes, there was some comfort in being around others.

MATT: That's what you need right now . . . you need to be around others. And when you are alone you should feel good about yourself and focus on how you've done the best you could throughout this ordeal.

Matt, albeit once again well intentioned in this exchange, has not focused on whether Claire has met her most basic physiological needs. It is not unusual to follow up with someone after an exchange like this, only to determine that the person is not doing as well as expected. From a Maslovian perspective, you have to establish a lower-order need, such as basic physiological requirements, before higher-order needs, such as affiliation and self-worth, can be established.

KEY POINT SUMMARY

1. As a constituent of the RAPID PFA model, psychological triage is prioritizing attendance to people according to their relative urgency of need for PFA and psychosocial support.

2. The specific criteria that determine urgency vary from person to person and situation to situation, but certain constants appear worth mentioning:
   a. Medical crises
   b. Maslovian physical needs (water, food, shelter)
   c. Safety
   d. Psychological/behavioral instability
      i. Tendencies for behavioral impulsivity
      ii. Diminished cognitive capabilities (insight, recall, problem solving), but most important a diminished ability to understand the consequences of one's actions
      iii. An acute loss of future orientation or a feeling of helplessness

   Survivors with unmet needs (items a–c) or survivors who manifest posttraumatic illness/dysfunction (item d, i–iii) would be considered as in need of urgent/higher-priority attention.

3. Predictors of posttraumatic illness/dysfunction include the following:
   a. Severity (Intensity × Chronicity) of trauma exposure
   b. Post-event-perceived guilt; negative appraisal of self
   c. Peritraumatic dissociation
   d. Peritraumatic depression
   e. Perceived life threat
   f. Prior psychiatric history, especially acute stress disorder or posttraumatic stress disorder

g. Lack of perceived social support

h. Seeing human remains

i. Head injury (concussion, traumatic brain injury)

4. Assessment and psychological triage should be seamlessly integrated. The figure included here represents that integration.

Figure 7.1   *Assessment* and *psychological triage* should be
seamlessly integrated

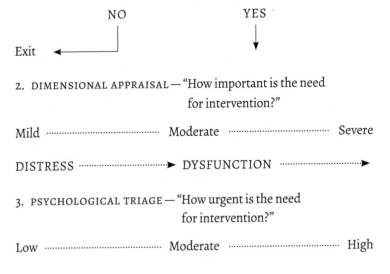

STEPS IN THE OVERALL DETERMINATION
OF THE NEED FOR INTERVENTION

1. BINARY SCREENING — "Is there any evidence of need for
PFA/psychosocial intervention?"

NO   YES

Exit ←

2. DIMENSIONAL APPRAISAL — "How important is the need
for intervention?"

Mild ················· Moderate ················· Severe

DISTRESS ···············► DYSFUNCTION ···············►

3. PSYCHOLOGICAL TRIAGE — "How urgent is the need
for intervention?"

Low ················· Moderate ················· High

References

Brewin, C. R., Andrews, B., & Valentine, J. D. (2000). Meta-analysis of risk factors for post-traumatic stress disorder in trauma-exposed adults. *Journal of Consulting and Clinical Psychology, 68*, 748–766. http://dx.doi.org /10.1037/0022-006x.68.5.748.

Everly, G. S., Jr. (1999). Toward a model of psychological triage. *International Journal of Emergency Mental Health, 1*, 151–154.

Everly, G. S., Jr., & Mitchell, J. T. (1999). *Critical incident stress management: A new era and standard of care in crisis intervention.* (2nd ed.). Ellicott City, MD: Chevron.

Everly, G. S., Jr., & Parker, C. (Eds.). (2005). *Mental health aspects of disaster: Public health preparedness and response.* Baltimore, MD: Johns Hopkins Bloomberg School of Public Health.

Kleim, B., Ehlers, A., & Glucksman, E. (2007). Early predictors of chronic post-traumatic stress disorder in assault survivors. *Psychological Medicine, 10*, 1457–1467. http://dx.doi.org/10.1017/S0033291707001006.

Lakein, A. (1973). *How to get control of your time and your life.* New York, NY: New American Library.

Maslow, A. H. (1970). *Motivation and personality.* New York, NY: Harper & Row.

McCabe, O. L., Everly, G. S., Jr., Brown, L. M., Wendelboe, A. M., Abd Hamid, N. H., Tallchief, V. L., & Links, J. M. (2014). Psychological first aid: A consensus-derived, empirically supported, competency-based training model. *American Journal of Public Health, 104*, 621–628. http://dx.doi.org/10.2105/AJPH.2013 .301219.

Ozer, E. J., Best, S. R., Lipsey, T. L., & Weiss, D. S. (2003) Predictors of post-traumatic stress disorder and symptoms in adults: A meta-analysis. *Psychological Bulletin, 129*, 52–73. http://dx.doi.org/10.1037/0033-2909.129 .1.52.

EIGHT | I—Intervention

Tactics to Stabilize and Mitigate Acute Distress

ASSESSMENT AND TRIAGE in the RAPID model, our previous two chapters, are not only a preface to this next stage of psychological intervention techniques intended to mitigate acute distress but also essential in formulating your intervention plan. Beginning interventionists are usually well trained in reflective listening techniques; thus, they understand the power of allowing, if not fostering, cathartic ventilation (i.e., expression of emotions). But they also understand that sometimes ventilative expression is not enough to mitigate intense distress or dysfunction. So, it is common for them to ask, "Other than just listening to their 'story,' how do I know what else to do to help this person?" The answer is largely revealed in the assessment and psychological triage phases—the guided conversation wherein the person in distress discusses some critical life event and the impact that event has had on him. Rather than leaving you to your own intuitive devices, we shall review a brief psychological pharmacopeia of sorts, a list of specific intervention tactics from which you may select one or many to assist a person in acute distress. Noted psychologist Theodore Millon and his colleagues asserted, "The palette of methods and techniques available to the [interventionist] must be commensurate with the idiographic heterogeneity of the [person] for whom the methods and techniques are intended" (Millon et al., 1999, p. 145). Let's take a look at intervention options.

Explanatory Guidance

People in distress often feel disempowered, even helpless. Therefore, one of the best things you can do as a crisis interventionist is to empower them. One of the most effective ways to empower someone is to give them information—knowledge about what happened to them, why it happened, and what reactions are common versus those that are not. This is called *explanatory guidance*.

Some common questions a person may ask in the wake of a traumatic event or in the midst of a posttraumatic reaction are "How did this happen?"; "Why am I reacting this way?"; "Why is this bothering me so much?"; or "What's happening to me?" In the absence of credible external information, people answer their own questions. Their answers are sometimes wrong or far more negative, even catastrophic, than is reality. Anticipate these questions as you listen to the story in the assessment phase. Prepare to answer questions, if possible, before they are asked. When you do not know the answer, say so, but direct the person to sources that can assist them.

Everly and Lating (2004) postulate that survivors often burden themselves with several psychological themes or interpretations. The person may not be aware that these themes are causing or, at least, fueling her current distress or dysfunction. These themes can be psychologically distressing or pathogenic after a critical incident, especially if the person in crisis becomes obsessional and unable to concentrate on anything other than these themes. However, when these themes, or assumptive errors, are identified interventionists can often begin to help people regain some sense of control. Here are some of the more common assumptive errors:

- Pathologizing what is often a normal and expected stress reaction (fight-or-flight response) to a disaster or trauma (see chapter 3). Here survivors unfamiliar with intense stress reactions of posttraumatic syndromes imagine the worst possible explanations and outcomes associated with their reactions.

- Guilt, albeit often self-imposed, for either making a mistake (doing something they should not have done) or not doing more to prevent something terrible from happening (not doing something that they should have done that might have been preventive or protective). This is especially common in emergency services personnel and the military. Given their training to take control in chaotic circumstances and the expectation on the part of everyone that this is what they will do, these personnel commonly take responsibility for things over which they had no actual control. Or they ceaselessly blame themselves when they do indeed make a mistake. (Be careful here *not* to blame people. Using a paraphrase, simply point out what they are doing, if it seems a recurrent theme. If the guilt seems unfounded you may respectfully and gradually employ cognitive reframing to offer an alternative explanation. More on this later.)

- Survivor guilt (blaming oneself for surviving when others did not).

- Incidents that violate one's belief in a just and fair world (e.g., "Why do bad things happen to innocent children?" or "Why do good people die young?"). Be careful not to offer a simple solution to a complex question. In general, resolution of this enigma is impossible. Gradual acceptance is most commonly the means to peace of mind.

- The belief that one's trust was betrayed (e.g., betrayal from someone or some group/organization once trusted). Betrayal from an intimate partner or confidant may be considered a form of trauma. Such a perceived betrayal is often expressed as feeling abandoned by others and is particularly salient when the perceived betrayal occurs from a source that is supposed to be trusted.

- Vicarious personal identification with some terrible event or some person who was a victim of some traumatic incident. This countertransference reaction results from a breakdown in the interpersonal or psychological space that separates listener from survivor.

As a crisis interventionist, your role is not to treat these issues, but there is often power in acknowledging them when asked the question, "Why do I feel this way?" (Abramson, Seligman, & Teasdale, 1978; Everly & Lating, 2004; Kamen & Seligman, 1989).

If such a theme is identified as particularly salient or even causative in determining the person's adverse reactions to an incident, then cognitive reframing, or a reinterpretation, may be useful in mitigating the reaction, over and above mere clarification. Cognitive reframing will be discussed later in this chapter.

Anticipatory Guidance

Anticipatory guidance is making the person in crisis aware of possible psychological or physical stress reactions that may be experienced within the next few hours or days postincident. This form of mental preparation serves to set appropriate expectations, thus reducing the chance that someone might decompensate in reaction to a normal pattern of posttraumatic distress. So, for example, you might say to someone:

"You might have some difficulty sleeping."

"Be aware that you may be more irritable than usual."

"It's pretty common to replay this incident over and over in your mind."

"People sometimes lose their appetite."

"Don't be surprised if you want to avoid going back to the area where the incident occurred."

"It's fairly common to withdraw and want to be left alone after an experience like this."

A counterpoint might be that by explaining certain reactions in advance you actually "cause" them by setting such expectations. Although there may indeed be a small chance that you cause certain reactions, the failure to warn someone of a potential reaction could result in a catastrophic self-interpretation. You must decide, depending on the individual's presentation, which risk is greater.

While both explanatory guidance and anticipatory guidance are means of providing reassurance and fostering hope, be careful not to dismiss someone's concerns or to normalize a serious reaction.

Cognitive Reframing

As humans, we desire to make sense or meaning out of the world around us. We don't like the unknown. We also like the perception of being in control of ourselves and of our environment. Because we generally agree that the world does not have intrinsic meaning, and to enhance our sense of control, we take information from our environments and infer meaning. According to psychologist Albert Bandura (1997), the primary factor underlying a stressful event is the individual's *perceived* inefficiency in coping with or controlling it. Therefore, how we perceive, interpret, and assign meaning to events will directly influence our emotions and behaviors (Nystul, 1999). You can see we have entered a far more subjective domain compared to explanatory and anticipatory guidance just reviewed.

This is an imposing concept, yet one that serves as the foundation of cognitive-behavioral therapy (CBT) (Beck, 1991; Meichenbaum, 1985). CBT emphasizes the use of verbal interventions that challenge irrational, unrealistic beliefs and help to modify ineffective behaviors as a way to improve functioning (Weiten, 2013). Albert Ellis (1995, 1999), a prominent psychologist who developed a theory known as rational emotive behavior therapy, believed that emotional disturbance results not from reality but from irrational thinking. Ellis is credited with saying, "Rational beliefs bring us closer to getting good results in the real world." To evoke a more pop-culture reference, albeit one that might possibly be somewhat dated for some, Bruce Lee, the renowned martial artist, is credited with a very similar construct by saying, "As you think, so shall you become." The message from both is that if we interpret events positively, we will usually feel better. Conversely, negative interpretations often lead to or exacerbate discomfort.

Let's now apply this theory in the aftermath of a traumatic event. Under considerable distress, we may not think clearly, let alone accurately. These inaccurate perspectives and unrealistic thoughts and interpretations about events often lead to misinterpretations, negative underlying beliefs, and misguided assumptions about what occurred. These thoughts left unchecked can negatively influence one's sense of self and self-worth. A crisis interventionist can assist in these instances by helping people identify these thoughts, evaluate how realistic or unrealistic they might be, and help them to change their inaccurate, or possibly distorted, thinking before negative underlying assumptions and beliefs become more embedded. Changing the meaning assigned to a situation or to oneself is known as cognitive reframing, or cognitive restructuring, and is a basic structural, applied tenet of CBT (Meichenbaum, 1985).

An example of an effective cognitive reframe that resonates with us occurred in an exchange between a peer support crisis interventionist and a firefighter. The firefighter had responded to a house fire in which one child survived and one child died. The firefighter berated himself because he did not locate the second child in time; the smoke was dense, and the child was hidden in a closet. After listening to the firefighter question his decision making and then himself for several minutes, the crisis interventionist said,

> I hear your sadness and the questioning of your responsibility in the loss of this child. And no doubt, that is a tragic and horrendous situation. But here's something for you to consider. If you had not been there, we would be dealing right now with the death of two children, not one. You didn't lose a life; that life was likely lost when you arrived. You *saved* a life. You saved a life. If you were not there, and if you did not respond the way you did, two lives would have been lost. When you're ready, maybe you can start thinking about what you did right instead of what you think you did wrong.

Cognitive reframing is a powerful tool for acute stabilization and mitigation. Just be careful not to argue with people. With time, they become more receptive to alternative interpretations of themselves and the critical incident. Consider using these types of cognitive re-frames, or alterations, if they seem warranted based on assessment:

- *Correction of errors in fact.* The conclusion the person reached is not supported by the facts. Respectfully point out that there are facts that would contradict their conclusion.
- *Disputing illogical thinking.* "I've heard what you've said, but I'm not following you." "It just doesn't make sense to me, but perhaps I'm missing something."
- *Challenging catastrophic* (the worst will always happen) *thinking.* People often dwell on the worst-case scenario, although possible worst cases seldom happen. You might consider pointing out the actual likelihood (probability) of a worst case actually happening. Even if it does occur, focus should be on moving beyond its consequences, if possible.
- *Finding something positive, a hidden benefit.* Is there any good that can come from this adversity?
- *Raise reasonable doubt.* Sometimes people in distress subjectively interpret events or outcomes in ways that are negative or condemning, with little supportive evidence. It's really a belief in their worst fears. Yet given that there is only partial support for their view, there will be room for doubt. The interventionist can point out the stress-inducing point of view could be correct, but it could be wrong as well. So, it becomes a matter of choice which perspective the person adopts. Raise reasonable doubt that the most toxic perspective is correct, especially in situations in which the truth will never be known.

Stress Management

Critical incidents engender stress. Stress management techniques are not only good lifestyle practices but also valuable crisis interventions as well. Let's take a look at a few considerations.

Crisis and traumatic stress interfere with sleep. Sleep, which is an intricate process whose essential purpose remains unknown, is, however, associated with health and well-being (Goldsmith & Casola, 2006; Horne, 2006; Vandekerckhove & Cluydts, 2010). It appears to be an essential constituent of recovery from both physical illness and excessive stress. For instance, research has shown that 17 to 19 hours without sleep produces motor performance impairment comparable with a blood alcohol level (BAL) of 0.05%, and after 20 to 25 hours without sleep, impaired performance was consistent with a BAL of 0.1% (Williamson & Feyer, 2000). According to the Sleep Foundation (Suni, 2011), adults should be getting around seven to nine hours of sleep per day. When natural sleep patterns cannot be practiced, brief naps may mitigate the effects of sleep deprivation.

Nutrients in the food we consume, their proportion to other nutrients, and our genetic predispositions influence how our body copes with stress. According to Mokdad et al. (2004, 2005), approximately 15.2% of all deaths in the United States are attributable to poor diet and lack of exercise. The US Department of Agriculture (2010) recommends that 45% to 65% of the human diet consists of carbohydrates (e.g., fruits, vegetables, milk, table sugar, honey, rice, wheat, barley, oats, peanuts, beans, and potatoes), 10% to 35% consists of proteins (e.g., eggs, beef, fish, soybeans), and 20% to 35% consists of fats (e.g., red meats, cheeses, whole milk, bacon, butter, chocolate, and nuts). In addition, and as will be noted in the scenario, caffeine consumption, whether in coffee, tea, or energy drinks, while considered safe for healthy adults in quantities of less than 400 milligrams per day (Doepker et al., 2018; Nawrot et al., 2003) can be detrimental when consumed in larger quantities. For example, it might be worth noting that a six-ounce cup of coffee typically has between 77 and 150 milligrams of caffeine (Griffiths, Juliano, & Chausmer, 2003) while the caffeine in energy drinks, which are typically sold in 16-ounce cans, is generally around 10 milligrams per ounce (Chen et al., 2019). So make sure those you are trying to assist are careful with consuming energy drinks.

One of the most effective combinations of intervention tactics to reduce stress in the aftermath of a critical incident is to foster one's perception of control while enhancing one's ability to cope or to manage the event. It is often advantageous as you provide psychological first aid (PFA) to ask, "What have you done in the past to help manage stressful situations?" This seemingly benign question provides the subtle yet affirming notion that the person in distress has handled daunting situations in the past. It is empowering. Moreover, it provides the framework for a beneficial problem-solving discussion of what specifically this person has done successfully in the past and how those strategies can be implemented now.

How one thinks about or interprets a situation can greatly affect its outcome. A foundational goal of cognitive-behavioral therapy is to challenge irrational appraisals and assumptions that can lead to emotional distress. From a practical perspective, cognitive reframing can help to reduce stress. One type of cognitive reframe, and one often associated with the emergency services culture to reduce stress, is humor. This, however, is sometimes in the form of gallows humor, which makes light of unpleasant, serious, or traumatic situations. This type of response, while potentially offensive to some, has been thought to be used by emergency responders as a way to affect their appraisal of traumatic events, to help them recover, and to foster social interactions (Abel, 2002; Martin, 2002). Therefore, as a PFA provider, be aware that you might hear the use of humor. However, as a provider you should be reluctant about ever initiating humor; instead, use it sparingly and cautiously in response to what you hear or observe in others.

We have tried to establish that changing the way one thinks can help to alter the way one feels. However, changing the way one feels physically (e.g., using relaxation techniques) can also help to alter the way one interprets events. Therefore, strategies that decrease physical arousal can be rewarding. During the intervention phase of the RAPID model, it is not prudent to try to teach sophisticated relaxation techniques, such as meditation, yoga, or active neuromuscular relaxation, because of time constraints. Also, a person in distress may experience cortical inhibition, which makes it challenging to teach intricate relaxation techniques. However, one technique we do recommend, if it seems appropriate, is to help the person control her breathing. Controlling one's breathing, often with deep, diaphragmatic breaths that oxygenate the lower third of the lungs, can help stimulate the parasympathetic response (Telles & Naveen, 2008) and foster relaxation. There are two primary benefits of teaching diaphragmatic breathing:

(1) if it is done properly your body will respond favorably by reducing stress arousal mechanisms associated with the sympathetic nervous system, and (2) it can be done pretty much anyplace at any time. To assist you in utilizing diaphragmatic breathing, we have included a step-by-step description of the method in the appendix.

The ongoing scenario will demonstrate that exercise is one of the best ways to burn up excess neurochemicals released in response to a traumatic event. But how can this be? Isn't exercise stressful? Indeed, it is, but it differs from the emotionally laden stress response that occurs from exposure to traumatic events, particularly if one remains inactive. During exercise, constituents of the stress response, such as release of lactic acid, free fatty acid, epinephrine, and the demand on the cardiovascular and cardiorespiratory systems, are used in a healthful, productive manner. The release of endorphins (the body's own pain-killers) during exercise helps to foster positive feelings (Dishman & O'Connor, 2009). After completion of exercise, the body experiences parasympathetic nervous system recovery (see chapter 3), including decreased muscle tension (McGuigan & Lehrer, 2007), and the long-term benefits of exercise include reduced risk for coronary heart disease (World Health Organization, 2009). According to the American College of Sports Medicine (2010), health benefits can be attained from 30 or more minutes of moderate-intensity exercise five days a week or 20 minutes of vigorous-intensity activity three days a week.

Everly and Lating (2019) have reviewed the major categories of stress management techniques with reviews of effectiveness and guidelines for implementation.

Instillation of a Future Orientation—Hope

In the wake of great personal adversity, people often lose hope. It is essential that you try to foster hope. Depression is characterized by feelings of hopelessness and helplessness. Helping empower survivors of adversity through information, anticipatory guidance, cognitive reframing, and stress management all foster hope. However, be careful not to offer false assurances or to be dismissive of people's concerns no matter how amplified by the situation.

Enlisting the Support of Family and Friends

In the book *Stronger*, Everly, Strouse, and McCormack (2015) conclude that interpersonal support when adversity and trauma strike may be the single most powerful factor to foster resilience. Enlisting the support of friends and family of those affected by adversity can be not only effective but also highly efficient as well. When using PFA, you should always ask what interpersonal resources the person in crisis has available and how they can be accessed. This becomes especially important in the next phase of the RAPID model.

Delay Making Any Life-Altering Decisions/Changes

It is counterproductive to "argue" with distressed individuals about how they should feel or think. Change is often a delicate process. When you encounter someone who is on the verge of a self-defeating action, or just a bad decision, one of the best things you can do, rather than argue, is to advocate a delay before making any important or life-changing decisions.

Faith-Based Interventions

No discussion of psychological intervention in the wake of extreme adversity and trauma would be complete with mentioning the role of faith-based PFA. Survey data indicate that 86% of Americans believe in God or a "universal spirit" (Gallup, 2014). According to the American Red Cross (2001) survey, after the 9/11 terrorist attacks, during times of trauma, 59% of respondents were likely to seek support from a spiritual counselor, compared to seeking assistance from their primary care physicians or mental health professionals.

The opportunity for faith-based interventions was formalized in the US military on July 29, 1775, by an act of the Continental Congress. At that time, Congress allowed for the creation of an organized military chaplaincy. The opportunity for faith-based intervention, of course, existed prior to that informally any time a member of the "flock" would seek guidance or support from anyone who held a position of pastoral leadership.

Recognizing the potential value for many in the wake of disaster, Everly (2000) formulated the notion of *pastoral crisis intervention* (PCI). PCI may be defined as the functional integration of the principles and practices of psychological crisis intervention and disaster mental health response with the principles and practices of faith-based pastoral care/support (adapted from Everly, 2000). By way of parallelism, as crisis intervention is to counseling and psychotherapy, pastoral crisis intervention is to pastoral counseling and pastoral psychotherapy.

In addition to the value of attendance and interpersonal support common to all forms of crisis intervention and PFA, faith-based intervention might employ scriptural education and insight, ventilative confession, prayer, faith-based social support networks, rituals and sacraments, belief in divine intervention/forgiveness, and the unique ethos of the faith-based interventionist.

Exploring the potential to harness the power of the faith-based community and integrate it with PFA, Lee McCabe and his colleagues trained faith-based leadership in communities in the mid-Atlantic and the central regions of the United States in RAPID PFA and community resilience building. He and his teams found that RAPID PFA and community networking were effective in building personal confidence and community resilience of those trained (McCabe et al., 2012; McCabe, Semon, Lating, et al., 2014; McCabe, Semon, Thompson, et al., 2014).

Recognizing the limitations of faith and spirituality as a PFA intervention, Everly (2007) argued that such interventions should only be used by those properly trained in chaplaincy or faith-based pastoral care. Furthermore, the interventions should only be used in the following situations:

1. Receptive expectations. The expectation/desire on the part of the person(s) in crisis for such responses as prayer, scriptural guidance, provision of sacraments, or rituals.

2. Receptive state of mind. While a person in crisis may not be expecting such interventions, he is open or psychologically receptive

to pastoral intervention. Argumentation, or debate, should be avoided in the acute crisis state. Such actions, such as arguing, tend to make the interventionist part of the problem, not part of the solution.

Faith-based intervention can be employed not only with primary survivors but also with family members, emergency response personnel, and observers, but the same guidelines listed above are applicable.

When In Doubt

When in doubt, ask what the person needs most at that time. For example, "I'm so sorry you've gone through this experience. What can I do for you right now? Or "What do you need most, right now?" If you believe the answer is not possible or in some way is deleterious, then simply indicate that it may not be viable right now and ask for other suggestions.

Caution

To avoid mistakes, consider these points:

1. Whatever interventions you choose to implement, you must be careful not to further disempower or infantilize a person who already believes he has few if any options, unless he is truly psychologically incapacitated and unable to help himself.
2. Don't make promises you can't keep.
3. Recognize and respect that no two people are the same. Varied people have varied ways to cope with stress. Some become introverted and analytic. Others become extroverted and highly cathartic. Some become angry. Some use denial and compartmentalize their experiences. Some use work as a distraction.
4. Don't assume someone needs intervention merely on the basis of exposure to a traumatic event alone.
5. Be careful not to interfere with another person's natural methods of resilience, as long as they are not injurious to themselves or to others.

Demonstration of the I in RAPID Model

Now that Matt has helped establish and prioritize that Claire is meeting her basic physiological needs, he can turn his focus to specific tactics to assist her. Part of this will entail revisiting some of the information he gathered through his assessment, but he will now provide more specific explanatory and anticipatory guidance, along with helping Claire to think about certain aspects of what occurred differently, continuing to instill hope, and providing stress management suggestions. Let's see how this progresses:

MATT, *crisis interventionist*: Good for you, Claire . . .I admire your resolve. I also realize how unlikely it is at this time that another tree will fall. But your concerns and reactions are understandable.

CLAIRE: Thanks. I'm glad you hear me.

MATT: I'm trying my best to listen to and hear everything you're saying. And what I'm particularly glad to hear is that you have a safe place to stay and that your sister will provide you with support. It's equally as good to know that you've been able to eat.

CLAIRE: Me too. It's a relief.

MATT: I also haven't forgotten some of the other signs of distress you were telling me about, and I wanted to talk more about them. Okay?

CLAIRE: I know I have far too much going on, don't I?

MATT: You've been through a traumatic event, and I just want you to know that before we talk more specifically about some of your reactions, given what you've been through, the reactions you've described thus far, while not comfortable, are actually normal.

CLAIRE: So, I'm not losing my mind?

MATT: You're *not* losing your mind.

CLAIRE: That's good to know.

MATT: In fact, given what you've experienced, I'd actually be more surprised if you were *not* displaying some of these signs of distress!

CLAIRE: Really?

MATT: Yes. Let's talk more about it. Is there a particular response that you're more concerned about right now?

CLAIRE: Hmm . . .Well, right now I'm mostly concerned about getting to sleep, and I was really bothered by the nightmares about trees falling—nightmares about trees . . .that seems kinda crazy, huh?

MATT: It's really not that unusual at all. Nightmares can certainly be frightening, but in situations like yours, it's often an indication of the emotional part of your brain trying to process information at a time when it's ready. And, for most of us, this is when we're sleeping. The frequency of nightmares usually decreases with time.

CLAIRE: Okay.

MATT: What have you tried in the past to help you to get to sleep?

CLAIRE: Well, in the past several years, there have been some occasions, maybe once or twice every other month, that I've used brandy at night to help me get to sleep.

MATT: Alcohol will often help you get to sleep, but it interferes with your quality of sleep. Mainly, it doesn't keep you asleep. Moreover, alcohol generally follows the same pathways in the brain that the stress response does. So, given that your brain right now is producing so many stress chemicals to keep you alert and active, you really don't need any other chemicals, like alcohol, being added to the mix.

CLAIRE: Hmm . . .that makes a lot of sense.

MATT: Do you drink alcohol at other times?

CLAIRE: I might have an occasional glass of wine with dinner, but that's only when I'm out with friends—maybe once a month.

MATT: Okay.

CLAIRE: So what can I do to help myself get to sleep?

MATT: Here are some suggestions. Make sure the room where you're trying to sleep is dark. So avoid having the television or computer screen on. Use some background noise, like soothing music or sounds of a waterfall, if that helps you to fall asleep. If you're not asleep in about 20 minutes, get up and do something boring until you feel sleepy again, like reading something technical. Another suggestion is to cover your clock or turn it in the other direction.

CLAIRE: Why's that?

MATT: Have you ever tried to sneak a peek at your alarm clock in the middle of the night, you know, with one eye, hoping that the clock won't "see you"?

CLAIRE, *chuckling*: Boy have I!

MATT: Well, alarm clocks are undefeated in staring contests!

CLAIRE, *lightly laughing*: I suppose they are!

MATT: Do you drink caffeine?

CLAIRE: I often have two cups of coffee in the morning, and then one, maybe two, diet colas in the afternoon.

MATT: Caffeine can cause sleep problems up to 12 hours after drinking it. So you might want to consider cutting back on it or even eliminating it after lunch, if you continue having trouble sleeping at night.

Also, when you sleep your body's internal temperature drops to its lowest level. Therefore, raising your body's temperature before going to sleep is thought by some to accelerate this cooling down process and to facilitate sleeping. So there might be some benefit for you to drink something warm and noncaffeinated and nonalcoholic about 20 minutes before going to bed. Moreover, taking a hot bath or shower about 45 minutes before going to bed might be helpful.

Last, you might want to avoid going to bed on a particularly full stomach because digestion can disrupt your sleep. But you also don't want to go to bed hungry. Good late-night snacks, which are high in carbohydrates, include a bowl of cereal and milk, bread, or crackers.

CLAIRE: These are very helpful suggestions. I'll try them.

MATT: Also, the other symptoms you described—not thinking clearly, having your hands being cold and clammy, your mouth being dry, and wanting to be left alone—are also typical reactions in the aftermath of what you've experienced.

However, I want to reiterate that just because they're common doesn't mean in any way that they don't matter or that they're comfortable.

CLAIRE: Thanks. Again, that's good to know.

MATT: Claire, I know it's only been a short time since the event, but are there any other signs or symptoms that you've experienced?

CLAIRE: I'm currently feeling an odd combination of fatigue and restlessness. But, as I said, I really didn't sleep last night.

MATT: You're right. It's not surprising that you feel some fatigue given your lack of sleep, and the restlessness is likely part of your nervous system working to protect you.

CLAIRE: Protect me?

MATT: Yeah, as I've alluded to, when we experience extreme stress our nervous system releases chemicals to keep us alert and to keep us going, in case our bodies need to respond actively and quickly. So this might explain why you're feeling a sense of fatigue but at the same time feeling restless.

CLAIRE: Huh!

MATT: It takes energy, in the form of food, to produce these chemicals. So it's good that you were able to eat this morning. And sometimes when people are stressed, they "forget" to eat, but remember nutrition is important.

CLAIRE: I'll keep that in mind.

MATT: Claire, there's no doubt that this is a challenging and stressful situation for you. I'm wondering, however, what have you done in the past to get yourself through stressful situations?

CLAIRE: When Jim started getting sicker, I would find comfort and support from my sister and friends. I also knew that it was important for me to keep busy. I had to keep busy. Sometimes I would live day to day, hour to hour, or even minute to minute . . . I had to keep occupied.

Also, Jim and I had a wonderful dog, Acorn, a yellow lab, and some of the most relaxing times I can recall were taking her for brisk walks in the morning and at dusk; there was something very soothing, almost peaceful about this. Acorn passed away about a year after Jim died. I miss the walks with her, and, you know, I haven't taken these walks since.

MATT: So it seems like social support, keeping busy, and exercising by taking walks with Acorn were all helpful?

CLAIRE: Yes.

MATT: Anything else?

CLAIRE: Hmm...well, in addition to the photo albums that were so important to me, I used to write in a journal on a regular basis, maybe every other night. It allowed me to have very personal time to collect and process my thoughts and feelings.

MATT: Claire, that sounds very powerful...and helpful for you. Anything else you can think of?

CLAIRE: Umm. Maybe it's not something that I did but something I didn't do.

MATT: Something you didn't do?

CLAIRE: Within days of Jim passing, I contacted a real estate agent to put the house on the market. I just didn't think I could live here anymore. However, my sister encouraged me to wait a while before making this decision. I'm glad I did. Even though things didn't turn out well a couple of days ago, I'm glad I kept our house.

MATT: What you're describing are really good strategies to help with a stressful time. Support from others has been shown time and time again to be one of the best things to help in the aftermath of traumatic events. Delaying making life-altering decisions, as you've noted, can be beneficial. And taking walks with your dog also was a great way to help with the stress response.

CLAIRE: Why's that?

MATT: As we talked about earlier, when we get stressed our bodies release chemicals to keep us alert and ready to perform. It takes energy to produce these chemicals, and it takes energy to burn them up. If we don't burn them up effectively, these chemicals can create a negative effect on our bodies. Over time, it's like they can become toxic. So we need to get rid of them, and the best way to do is by...

CLAIRE: Let me guess—exercising?

MATT: Exercising! And what's one of the first things we give up when we get stressed?

CLAIRE: Exercising.

MATT: Exercising!

CLAIRE: Hmm. So, Acorn was helping me out in ways I never even knew.

MATT: Indeed, she was. Do you regularly exercise now?

CLAIRE: Mostly by gardening a couple times a week for about one hour, but my sister has a dog who loves to walk, and I could take him for walks in the morning and at night when I'm staying with her.

MATT: That sounds like a really helpful idea.

CLAIRE: And even when her dog is unavailable, like when my home here is rebuilt, or if I move somewhere else, I could still take walks on my own.

MATT: Sure. And the journaling you used to do might be helpful now as well. Studies have shown the benefit of how cathartic writing can be, and it doesn't have to be for a long time, maybe just 20 minutes a day about your reactions, emotions, and feelings.

CLAIRE: I found it helpful years ago, and I hope to find some of the journals that were in my basement. I'd like to read what I used to write.

MATT: I hope they help if you find them. They might be very inspirational.

CLAIRE: I've been through a lot in my life, but I've always been optimistic.

MATT: It certainly seems that you have been through a lot, and this current experience seems particularly daunting. But your optimism is very encouraging to hear.

CLAIRE: My grandmother used to say, "This, too, shall pass," and I believe that. I also find tremendous comfort in my faith. And although I don't want to stay at the church right now, I find peace and comfort knowing it's there and can see myself spending more time there over the next several weeks, if not several months, or more.

MATT: Faith can certainly be very important during times of distress, and it sounds like this could be a wonderful resource for you. It also seems that the support you'll get from your sister, your daughter, your son-in-law, your granddaughter, and your neighbors will be beneficial.

CLAIRE: I really believe they will.

MATT: It seems like you have a lot of people in your corner offering support.

CLAIRE: I'm likely going to need them.

MATT: What else can I do for you right now?

CLAIRE: You allowed me to talk, and that's been so helpful. But now I really feel like I need to spend some time sorting through what's left. I hope to be able to salvage some material things of value.

Scenario Summary

Matt's recall of some of the signs and symptoms that Claire presented earlier demonstrates how he was listening to her, hearing her, and gathering information. It was appropriate and likely reassuring for Claire who was slightly catastrophizing (thinking that another tree might fall, that she was losing her mind, or that her nightmares were a reflection that she was crazy) that Matt provided a general sense of normalization early on in this intervention exchange. Compare this to the possible mistake noted in the assessment phase scenario when the crisis interventionist was overly eager and repetitive in trying to normalize almost everything that Claire disclosed. In this exchange, Matt also allowed Claire to prioritize that getting to sleep and nightmares were her current primary concerns. Matt used explanatory guidance, anticipatory guidance, as well as problem solving to address these and other issues he assessed, such as caffeine consumption and eating. He also was able to use a subtle and apparently acceptable smattering of humor (staring at the alarm clock) that Claire responded favorably to hearing. Although he provided a lot of input and suggestions, Matt remained present and allowed Claire to talk.

Asking Claire about what she has done to handle stressful situations in her past seemed to be both empowering for her and provided her with several good stress management strategies, including her need to exercise, her success journaling in the past, the benefits she discovered by delaying important decisions, and the strength she has found from her faith. Matt will use this information to continue to incorporate her responses and to infuse other aspects of intervention covered in this chapter when we highlight *disposition* in the scenario in chapter 9.

Mistakes to Avoid

Everyone is different, and you want to meet people where they are. Do not argue with someone, overpathologize what's presented, minimize their concerns, or offer false promises. The following exchange demonstrates why:

CLAIRE: That's good to know.

MATT: In fact, given what you've experienced, I'd actually be more surprised if you were not displaying some of these signs of distress!

CLAIRE: Really?

MATT: Yes. Take, for example, the nightmares. Your brain is trying to sort through the event, and I can assure you that it will. It just needs a little more time.

CLAIRE: How long?

MATT: Oh, I don't know for sure, but I'd say a week . . .tops. By the way, what have you done in the past to get yourself to sleep?

CLAIRE: Well, I don't like to admit it, but I've used alcohol in the past to help me get to sleep.

MATT: Alcohol . . .hmm (*five-second pause*). Do you have a drinking problem?

CLAIRE: A drinking problem? Why, heavens, no. What would make you think that?

MATT: Sometimes people deny having a drinking problem. Do you ever drink alcohol in the mornings?

CLAIRE: No! I drink a glass or two of brandy maybe once every other month to help me sleep. It's not a problem, and I'm sorry now that I mentioned it. Can we talk about something else, please?

MATT: I'm sorry, I didn't mean to offend you. The last thing I will say about it is that if it is a problem, you really should get some help.

This is an extreme example of what could occur if the PFA provider makes false promises (such as when the nightmares will end), over-pathologizes, and becomes argumentative. As PFA providers, we all bring our personal histories, temperaments, and life experiences to any RAPID encounter. Matt's reaction and current line of questioning in this scenario might lead one to question that he might have some type of connection or possible history with substance use.

Faith-based interventions in the aftermath of a disaster can be very powerful. However, they should only be employed by those trained in chaplaincy or faith-based pastoral care. Consider, for example, the potential awkwardness of the following exchange:

CLAIRE: I also find tremendous comfort in my faith. And although I don't want to stay at the church, I find peace and comfort knowing it's there and can see myself spending more time there over the next several weeks.

MATT: You probably should Claire. If what happened is indeed part of God's will, it might be important for you to explore this, particularly if you become more and more preoccupied about the loss.

The crisis interventionist, who has likely not been trained in pastoral crisis care, is stepping outside his training and boundaries with his suggestion that what happened to Claire was part of God's will. For those not trained in pastoral crisis intervention, it is better to try to normalize that the person is having the response than it is to try and interpret it.

KEY POINT SUMMARY

It takes skill to choose the right intervention at the right time for the right person(s) in a crisis or disaster situation. Commonly used tactics (mechanisms of action) intended to mitigate acute distress and dysfunction include the following:

1. Meet basic medical and physical needs (cf. Maslow, 1970)
2. Cathartic ventilation
3. Explanatory guidance—education, normalization (as appropriate)
4. Anticipatory guidance
5. Distraction (tasks or conversation; usually more of a stabilization technique)
6. Cognitive reframing
   a. Correction of errors in fact
   b. Disputing illogical thinking
   c. Challenging catastrophic thinking
   d. Finding something positive, a hidden benefit
   e. Raise reasonable doubt
7. Stress management
   a. Sleep
   b. Nutrition
   c. Relaxation techniques
   d. Exercise
8. Instillation of a future orientation—hope
9. Delay making any life-altering decisions/changes
10. Enlisting the support of family and friends (although this is also a tactic used in the final stage of the RAPID model)
11. Faith-based intervention
12. When in doubt, ask what the person needs most now. For example, "I'm so sorry you've gone through this experience. What can I do for you right now?" or "What do you need most, right now?"

And never underestimate the power of merely being "present" to support another human being during, or in the wake of, adversity. Whatever tactics you do choose to employ, always be careful not to disrupt a person's natural trajectory of resilience.

References

Abel, M. H. (2002). Humor, stress, and coping strategies. *Humor: International Journal of Humor Research, 15*, 365–381. http://dx.doi.org/10.1515/humr.15.4.365.

Abramson, L. Y., Seligman, M. E. P., & Teasdale, J. D. (1978). Learned helplessness in humans: Critique and reformulation. *Journal of Abnormal Psychology, 87*, 49–74. http://dx.doi.org/10.1037/0021-843x.87.1.49.

American College of Sports Medicine. (2010). *ACSM's guidelines for exercise testing and prescription* (8th ed.). Philadelphia, PA: Lippincott Williams & Wilkins.

American Red Cross. (2001). *The ripple effect*. Alexandria, VA: American Red Cross.

Bandura, A. (1997). *Self-efficacy: The exercise of control*. New York, NY: W. H. Freeman.

Beck, A. T. (1991). Cognitive therapy: A 30-year retrospective. *American Psychologist, 46*, 368–337. http://dx.doi.org/10.1037/0003-066x.46.4.368.

Chen, X., Liu, Y., Jaenicke, E. C., & Rabinowitz, A. N. (2019). New concerns on caffeine consumption and the impact of potential regulations: The case of energy drinks. *Food Policy, 87*, 101746. http://dx.doi.org/10.1016/j.foodpol.2019.101746.

Dishman, R. K., & O'Connor, J. P. (2009). Lessons in exercise neurobiology: The case of endorphins. *Mental Health Physical Activity, 2*, 4–9. http://dx.doi.org/10.1016/j.mhpa.2009.01.002.

Doepker, C., Franke, K., Myers, E., Goldberger, J. J., Liberman, H. R., O'Brien, C., . . .Wikoff, D. (2018). Key findings and implications of a recent systematic review of the potential adverse effects of caffeine consumption in healthy adults, pregnant women, adolescents, and children. *Nutrients, 10*, 1536. http://dx.doi.org/10.3390/nu10101536.

Ellis, A. (1995). Rational-emotive behavior therapy. In R. Corsini (Ed.), *Current psychotherapies* (5th ed., pp. 162–196). Itasca, IL: F. E. Peacock.

Ellis, A. (1999). Why rational-emotive therapy to rational emotive behavior therapy? *Psychotherapy, 36*, 154–159. http://dx.doi.org/10.1037/h0087680.

Everly, G. S., Jr. (2000). Pastoral crisis intervention: Toward a definition. *International Journal of Emergency Mental Health, 2*, 69–71.

Everly, G. S., Jr. (2007). *Pastoral crisis intervention*. Ellicott City, MD: Chevron.

Everly, G. S., Jr., & Lating, J. M. (2004). *Personality-guided treatment of post-traumatic stress disorder.* Washington, DC: American Psychological Association.

Everly, G. S., Jr., & Lating, J. M. (2019). *A clinical guide to the treatment of the human stress response* (4th ed.). New York, NY: Springer Nature.

Everly, G. S., Jr., Strouse, D. A., & McCormack, D. (2015). *Stronger.* New York, NY: AMACOM.

Gallup. (2014). Religion. http://www.gallup.com/poll/1690/religion.aspx.

Goldsmith, J. R., & Casola, P. G. (2006). The basics for psychiatrists: An overview of sleep, sleep disorders, and psychiatric medications' effects on sleep. *Psychiatric Annals, 36,* 833–840.

Griffiths, R. R., Juliano, L. M., & Chausmer, A. L. (2003). Caffeine: Pharmacology and clinical effects. In A. W. Graham, T. K. Schultz, M. F. Mayo-Smith, R. K. Ries, & B. B. Wilford (Eds.), *Principles of addiction medicine* (3rd ed., pp. 193–224). Chevy Chase, MD: American Society of Addiction.

Horne, J. (2006). *Sleepfaring: A journey through the science of sleep.* New York: NY: Oxford University Press.

Kamen, L. P., & Seligman, M. E. P. (1989). Explanatory style and health. In M. Johnston & T. Marteau (Eds.), *Applications in health psychology* (pp. 73–84). New Brunswick, NJ: Transaction.

Martin, R. A. (2002). Is laughter the best medicine? Humor, laughter, and physical health. *Current Directions in Psychological Science, 11,* 216–220.

Maslow, A. H. (1970). *Motivation and personality.* New York, NY: Harper & Row.

McCabe, O. L., Marcum, F., Mosley, A., Gwon, H. S., Langlieb, A., Everly, G. S., Jr., . . .Links, J. M. (2012). Community capacity-building in disaster mental health resilience: A pilot study of an academic/faith partnership model. *International Journal of Emergency Mental Health, 14,* 112–124.

McCabe, O. L., Semon, N. L., Lating, J. M., Everly, G. S., Jr., Perry, C. J., Moore, S. S., . . .Links, J. M. (2014). An academic-government-faith partnership to build disaster mental health preparedness and community resilience. *Public Health Reports, 129*(Suppl 4), 96–106. http://dx.doi.org/10.1177/003335 49141296S413.

McCabe, O. L., Semon, N. L., Thompson, C. B., Lating, J. M., Everly, G. S., Jr., Perry, C. J., . . .Links, J. M. (2014). Building a national model of public mental health preparedness and community resilience: Validation of a dual-intervention, systems-based approach. *Disaster Medicine and Public Health Preparedness, 8,* 511–526. http://dx.doi.org/10.1017/dmp.2014.119.

McGuigan, F. J., & Lehrer, P. M. (2007). Progressive relaxation: Origins, principles, and clinical applications. In P. M. Lehrer, R. L. Woolfolk, & W. E.

Sime (Eds.), *Principles and practices of stress management* (3rd ed., pp. 57–87). New York, NY: Guilford Press.

Meichenbaum, D. (1985). *Stress innoculation training.* New York, NY: Pergamon.

Millon, T., Grossman, S., Meagher, D., Millon, C., & Everly, G. S., Jr. (1999). *Personality-guided therapy.* New York, NY: Wiley.

Mokdad, A. H., Marks, J. S., Stroup, D. F., & Gerberding, J. L. (2004). Actual causes of death in the United States, 2000. *Journal of the American Medical Association, 291,* 1238–1245. http://dx.doi.org/10.1001/jama.291.10.1238.

Mokdad, A. H., Marks, J. S., Stroup, D. F., & Gerberding, J. L. (2005). Correction: Actual causes of death in the United States, 2000 [Letter to the editor]. *Journal of the American Medical Association, 293,* 293–294. http://dx.doi.org/10.1001/jama.293.3.293.

Suni, E. (2011). How much sleep do we really need? Sleep Foundation, updated March 10, 2021. http://www.sleepfoundation.org/how-sleep-works/how-much-sleep-do-we-really-need.

Nawrot, P., Jordan, S., Eastwood, J., Rotstein, J., Hugenholtz, A., & Feeley, M. (2003). Effects of caffeine on human health. *Food Additives & Contaminants, 20,* 1–30. http://dx.doi.org/10.1080/0265203021000007840.

Nystul, M. S. (1999). *Introduction to counseling: An art and science perspective.* Boston, MA: Allyn and Bacon.

Telles, S., & Naveen, K. V. (2008). Voluntary breath in yoga: Its relevance and physiological effects. *Biofeedback, 36,* 70–73.

US Department of Agriculture. (2010). *Report of the Dietary Guidelines Advisory Committee on the dietary guidelines for Americans.* http//www.cnpp.usda.gov/Publications/Dietary Guidelines/2010/DGAC/Report/2010DGAC Report-camera-ready-Jan 11-11.pdf.

Vandekerckhove, M., & Cluydts, R. (2010). The emotional brain and sleep: An intimate relationship. *Sleep Medicine Reviews, 14,* 219–226. http://dx.doi.org/10.1016/j.smrv.2010.01.002.

Weiten, W. (2013). *Psychology: Themes and variations* (9th ed.). Belmont, CA: Wadsworth Cengage Learning.

Williamson, A. M., & Feyer, A. M. (2000). Moderate sleep deprivation produces impairments in cognitive and motor performance equivalent to legally prescribed levels of alcohol intoxication. *Occupational and Environmental Medicine, 57,* 649–655. http://dx.doi.org/10.1136/oem.57.10.649.

World Health Organization. (2009). *Global health risks: Mortality and burden of disease attributable to selected major risks.* Geneva, Switzerland: World Health Organization.

NINE

D—Disposition

Facilitating Access to Continued Care

DISPOSITION may be thought of as an attitude or general state of being. The disposition phase of the RAPID model is the final phase of the crisis intervention process. McCabe et al. (2014, p. 624) refer to this phase as "referral, liaison, and advocacy" and it is listed as a core competency. The need for this stage was underscored from the earliest discussions of psychological first aid (PFA) (American Psychiatric Association, 1954; Raphael, 1986). The goal of the disposition phase is to answer the question that is always pondered, if not verbally expressed, "So, where do we go from here?" The question is neither trite nor should it be taken lightly. Other than for a follow-up contact or two if possible, your interaction with any given survivor has ended when the steps in the RAPID model have been completed. So this phase becomes an important process by which you wrap up the interaction and make plans for next steps.

Where Do We Go From Here?

The disposition phase follows the intervention phase wherein you employed various acute state-dependent mechanisms of action in an attempt to mitigate acute distress and dysfunction, not cure the problem! It is common to ask the other person, "So, how are you feeling?" or "How are you doing right now?" The crisis interventionist must listen closely, integrate what was said with what has been observed, and then decide the next steps.

"Where do we go from here?" The answer is not as difficult as it may seem if you keep in mind the overarching goals of the RAPID model and the crisis intervention tactics:

1. Meet basic needs.
2. Stabilize acute psychological and/or behavioral reactions.
3. Mitigate acute distress, impairment, or dysfunction to assist in recovery of some degree of adaptive functionality.
4. Foster natural coping mechanisms.
5. Facilitate access to continued support, or higher-level care, if indicated.

On the basis of the assessment and psychological triage phases of the RAPID model, you formulated your plans on how best to assist the person in crisis. You employed whatever mechanisms of action you felt most appropriate throughout the interaction and especially in the intervention phase. Now you must determine the best next steps to take on this person's behalf, given the goals enumerated earlier. For example:

1. After your intervention, if the person seems more capable of taking care of herself or capable of discharging her responsibilities, then your intervention has ended. It is then recommended that you follow up with the person at a time deemed most appropriate. Sometimes a second follow-up may be useful. However, if a third follow-up seems indicated, it's probably time to facilitate access to another level of care.
2. After your intervention, if the person seems more capable of taking care of himself and capable of discharging his responsibilities but some form of informal support (friends, family, coworkers) would

be helpful, you can then serve to connect the person with those resources. Once again a follow-up may be useful.

3. After your intervention, if it is determined that the person cannot function independently or requires significant and more formalized support from others (psychological, medical, logistical, financial, spiritual), then facilitate access to further support (referral), serving as a liaison or perhaps even an advocate for the person (cf. McCabe et al., 2014).

Encouragement

A big challenge associated with the disposition phase is encouraging people to seek further support. They are often hesitant because they might believe accepting further assistance is a sign of weakness or may be stigmatizing. At this point, it is often helpful to remind them that seeking further assistance may be a means of helping those who depend on them more than a form of direct assistance for them. Sometimes the timing is simply not right. Therefore, it may be advisable to follow up after a reasonable time and offer to facilitate access to continued care.

In some instances, you may have to immediately request further assistance over objections to the contrary. Suicidal ideation, homicidal ideation, psychotic behavior, or any behavior that reaches the threshold of reckless endangerment to themselves or others would warrant further if not immediate assistance.

Resources

The resources available for further psychosocial support in the wake of adversity vary greatly. Friends, family, and coworkers are possibilities. Workplace-based employee assistance programs (EAP) can be extremely effective resources, especially if the EAP counselors have received specialized crisis intervention training. Walk-in general crisis centers, hospital emergency departments, houses of worship, crisis-oriented chaplaincy programs, non-EAP workplace resources (such as union-based services), and specialized crisis centers (domestic violence, rape crisis, drug overdose, veterans' crisis centers and hotlines, etc.) may also be considered. Calling 911 for law enforcement and/or paramedical support can be options as well. Disaster relief services (local, state, and national) will be an obvious choice in the wake of a natural disaster. The Salvation Army, the American Red Cross, and a host of other nongovernmental organizations respond to most disasters in the United States. After federally declared disasters, behavioral health resources associated with the Federal Emergency Management Agency and the Substance Abuse and Mental Health Services Administration are available. Decide next steps after consulting with the person in crisis on a case-by-case basis.

Familiarize yourself with the various state and national disaster response resources, as well as local crisis resources. Look into the response capacities of the state affiliates of the National Volunteer Organizations Active in Disaster.

Demonstration of the **D** in RAPID Model

The disposition phase of the RAPID process can be critically important to summarize the main points of the interaction, to assess how the person is currently doing, to delineate what the next steps for the person might be, and to make plans for follow-up. Matt's rapport with Claire and his ongoing assessment, prioritization, and intervention suggestions were relatively successful in stabilizing Claire's psychological and behavioral reactions, helping her to mitigate distress and providing her with several strategies to begin to move forward. Let's see how Matt ends the current RAPID exchange with Claire in the disposition scenario:

MATT, *crisis interventionist*: That sounds like a good plan.

CLAIRE: I just hope I can do it.

MATT: Claire, you've been through tough times before, and in addition to the support you received from others and your faith, you used effective strategies like exercising and journaling. Add to this now, ways to help sleep better and eat better, and you have a good plan to deal with what lies ahead.

CLAIRE, *after 10 seconds of silence*: What's that song . . . "the sun will come out, tomorrow" *(Claire makes a light-hearted attempt to sing the phrase and smiles warmly)*. It's just hard right now . . . really hard.

MATT: I can only imagine how hard this is right now, Claire. But optimism, your acknowledged faith, and the plans you have in place will help get you through these tough times.

CLAIRE: Spending time with you has helped to make it better for me. Thank you, Matt.

MATT: You're welcome, Claire. I'm so sorry you're going through this experience.

CLAIRE: I can really tell that you are.

MATT: I will be around for the next week or so at least. Would it be all right if I check in with you just to see how you are doing?

CLAIRE: Please do.

MATT: I certainly will. Would you be comfortable exchanging cell phone numbers? I realize I might see you out here, but would it be okay if I call you tomorrow around this time?

CLAIRE: Sure. Thanks, again. Here's my number.

Scenario Summary

Matt provided Claire with encouragement, hope, and support, and his summary of the main points of the suggestions he and Claire discussed seems to be an effective way to wrap up the current encounter. Claire seems to be displaying the expected amount and types of distress associated with her unexpected loss. There is no apparent need to refer her to a higher level of care at this time, but it can remain an option. The follow-up over the next couple of days will provide a valuable opportunity to further assess how she's doing and to determine whether other steps or level of care are warranted.

Mistakes to Avoid

It can be helpful in the disposition stage of the RAPID model to foster an expectation of success. However, consider what happens in the following exchange:

MATT: That sounds like a good plan.

CLAIRE: I just hope I can do it.

MATT: Oh, I promise that you can!

CLAIRE: A promise, huh . . . I just hope I don't disappoint you.

MATT: I don't see how you could. But on the remote chance you need some additional help, here's my number.

CLAIRE: I hope I don't feel like I need to use it.

MATT: I don't believe you will.

CLAIRE: How will I know?

MATT: You'll know.

Matt was attempting to foster hope and the expectation of success for Claire. However, compared to the previous disposition scenario, he did not provide a summary of their interaction in order to help solidify his rationale for this expectation. Even more egregious, and likely as a result of his belief that she needed no additional help, the crisis interventionist did not arrange for follow-up. Instead, he put the onus, without explanation or direction, on Claire to contact him if needed. This should not be done. The crisis interventionist should always make provisions and take the lead in facilitating follow-up, whether this is in person, over the phone, or electronically.

Follow-Up and Disposition

Although every RAPID encounter is different, the progression of what we provided throughout this scenario reflects what could occur in a typical, successful PFA encounter. However, not every RAPID encounter flows smoothly, and most of the questions PFA providers in training ask have to do with the rare but more challenging encounters.

To help facilitate exposure to these occurrences, we will now present three different follow-up scenarios that will require very different reactions and dispositional tactics from the crisis interventionist.

Scenario 1 Follow-Up

June 13: The crisis interventionist called Claire the next day as promised. Matt asked how she was doing and when she would return to the house. They agreed to meet the following day at 11:00 a.m.

June 14, 11:00 a.m.: Matt drives back to the site where Claire's house had been. Claire appears busy, looking through the rubble and is periodically placing personal belongings in boxes. It's a clear, sunny day, with a mild breeze blowing.

MATT: Hi, Claire!

Claire stands up and waves to Matt as she walks toward him.

CLAIRE: Oh, hi, Matt!

They are meeting one another on what is now a much emptier yard. The tree has been removed. They shake hands and then Claire gently hugs him.

MATT: So, how's it going?

Claire initiates a slow walk as she begins speaking. Matt walks alongside.

CLAIRE: You know, I've been sleeping better the last two nights. No nightmares. The tips you gave me have been helpful. No staring contests with the clock. And when I found I couldn't get to sleep, I got out of bed after about 20 minutes, went downstairs, and read some rather dull book before I returned to bed. I was asleep within minutes.

MATT: That's good to hear.

CLAIRE: Oh, and I've taken my sister's dog for a walk several times the past two days and nights. It's been very helpful, particularly when my sister joins us. I try to walk at a brisk pace.

MATT: It's good to have the support, and the exercise helps to burn up the excess neurochemicals. How have you been eating?

CLAIRE: I forgot to mention to you the other day, but my sister is a great cook, so, like before when I first spoke with you, no issues there.

MATT: That's good to hear. How is the searching through the debris progressing?

CLAIRE: I've found a few of my things, but I haven't found any of the photo albums. But you know something, the more I search for these things, the more I think that's all they are—just things. Maybe I'd feel differently if I find one of the albums. But for now, when I do find something, no matter how small, that was either mine, Jim's, or Marissa's, I feel excited, though the feeling fades quickly. So, I keep looking and I find something else, then I get a glimmer of excitement for a couple of seconds, and I put it in one of the boxes. But for what?! Do you understand what I mean? I realize I'm not upset about losing my *things*.

Claire pauses and appears to be searching for the right words. Sensing her apparent difficulty, Matt tries to assist her.

MATT: Claire, it seems like there have been some real ups and downs for you over the past couple of days. As you look back, what do you think the worst part of this ordeal has been for you thus far?

Claire stops walking and turns to face Matt. She speaks in a low, even, and thoughtful tone.

CLAIRE: I've lost another part of my life . . . I've lost memories. I've lost the things that remind me of Jim, Marissa, and the other people who were in some way a part of the house. I know that a house can be rebuilt. The insurance company so far has been very helpful in working with me. And, of course, I can buy new *things*, but for now, the ones that were lost were keeping different moments alive . . . what I had felt and who I had been with were kept alive . . . the sounds, the smells, the feel of what this home meant to me. But without the things that tie me to those memories, I'm afraid I might end up forgetting.

MATT: Are you saying that what is making this so painful right now is the fear that you will lose the memories of the people you loved?

CLAIRE: Yeah. That's right. That's what I'm afraid of.

MATT: Claire, I can imagine that the thought of losing those memories is frightening, and I clearly think you should keep searching for cherished items. But as precious as this house has been, and for what it meant for you and Jim to work together on it and to raise Marissa there, have you thought that the memories of those you love are not *in* those items? They are in your mind and in your heart. And no storm can ever take that away.

It was interesting to hear you the other day keep referring to the house as "our" house, and I'm assuming that you meant yours, Jim's, and Marissa's. As long as you maintain the memories in your mind and heart, the house can always be "our" house.

CLAIRE, *smiles*: Thanks, Matt.

MATT: Claire, I think you're doing really well to not only maintain your perspective but to try to work to grow from your experience. You seem very resilient. And I don't see a reason for that to change. However, if it's okay with you, I'd like to share the contact information for the free local counseling service that has been set up as a result of the disaster. Not that I expect that you'll need it, but if you find that you're not sleeping well or if your mood changes, or if something else unexpected occurs, then it might be helpful to have the resource so you can talk with someone about how you're doing. Would you please consider giving them a call if you find that you're not doing as well as you'd like?

CLAIRE: I hear what you're saying, and although I don't think I'll need it, I appreciate the backup and will call if needed.

MATT: And if you don't mind, I'd like to check in with you in the next couple of days just to see how you're doing.

CLAIRE: I would definitely appreciate that.

Scenario 1 Follow-Up Summary

The two-day passage of time is helpful in allowing Matt to assess further Claire's sleeping, eating, and exercising since they first met. She reports doing well. He also helped her with cognitively reframing

how she was considering the loss of the items in the home. As Matt
noted, the memories and value are in her mind and in her heart, and
not necessarily in the material items themselves. Reframing intervention provided at follow-up might stay with Claire and help her as she
progresses. In addition, and as noted in R phase of the RAPID scenario, Matt's ability to recall how Claire initially used the word *our* when
describing the loss may be considered part of the art of doing PFA.
Making these types of connections is not meant to be prescriptive in
doing the RAPID model, but sometimes when you're doing PFA you
hear something that sticks with you. It either seems inconsistent with
what the person is saying or it resonates with you at a cognitive or an
emotional level. Don't dismiss your gut-level feelings; there might be
a time and appropriate place later in the process for doing follow-up
to make this type of connection with someone. Last, Matt offered encouragement and expectations about her doing well but still offered
additional resources in case Claire needed them. She seemed to accept
them with the intention in which they were provided.

Mistakes to Avoid

In this scenario, Claire struggles with trying to find the connection
between the meaning attached to the lost items and her fear of losing memories of her loved ones. Matt uses reflective statements and
open-ended questions to allow her to speak more. Consider, instead,
the following exchange:

CLAIRE: I've found a few of my things, but I haven't found any of
the photo albums. But you know something, the more I search for
these things, the more I think that's all they are . . . things. Maybe
I'd feel differently if I found one of the albums. But, for now, when
I find something, no matter how small, that was either mine, Jim's,
or Marissa's, I feel excited, though the feeling fades quickly. So,
I keep looking, and I find something else, then I get a glimmer of
excitement for a couple of seconds, and I put it in one of the boxes.
But for what?! Do you understand what I mean? I realize I'm not
upset about losing my *things*.

MATT: You shouldn't be upset about losing things. Things can be replaced. And as I asked earlier, you have insurance to replace a lot of these things, right? And maybe if you find the albums you'll feel better.

Matt doesn't provide Claire with the opportunity to expand on what she's trying to find words to say. Similar to the possible mistakes to avoid noted in chapter 5 on reflective listening, Matt did not use reflective statements and returned to information that might not be relevant at this time (e.g., insurance). Moreover, by not doing this and responding so quickly, he misses the opportunity to help her with a possibly poignant cognitive reframe.

Another possible mistake to avoid is how Matt presents the information about a possible referral if Claire needs it. Consider the following exchange:

MATT: Claire, although I think you're doing well, and I'm really glad to hear that, I'd like to share the contact information for the free local counseling service in case you need to give them a call.

CLAIRE: You just said I'm doing well, and I feel like I'm doing okay given all that I've been through. So, why would I need to call a counseling service? Is there something I'm missing?

MATT: No, not at all. I just routinely give this out in case someone needs it.

CLAIRE: How would I know if I need it?

Although Matt was well intentioned, he did not provide enough context or establish the parameters around which providing this information made sense to Claire.

Scenario 2 Follow-Up

By the end of the previous scenario, Claire reported doing reasonably well, and Matt offered her some counseling resources if she believed they might be warranted in the future. However, given the exchange, this seemed unlikely if not unwarranted. However, consider how you might respond if, instead, this follow-up exchange with Claire occurred:

> *June 14, 11:00 a.m.: The crisis interventionist drives back to the site where Claire's house had been. Claire appears preoccupied and is staring at the debris. It's a clear, sunny day, with a mild breeze blowing.*

MATT: Hi, Claire!

CLAIRE, *quietly and with very little inflection in her voice*: Hello, Matt.

MATT: How are you doing?

CLAIRE: I hope I can give you the honest answer?

MATT: Of course, you can.

CLAIRE: Then, not well. Not well at all!

MATT: Claire, I'm so sorry to hear this. What's going on?

CLAIRE: When I went to my sister's, she didn't tell me that when she went to check on the water in her basement, she slipped on the steps and fell. As a result, she bruised her hip badly and twisted her ankle. I feel just awful for her, and I'm certainly willing to help, but it's been exhausting for me. I need to do all the cooking, wait on her, and the poor thing, she's in a lot of pain and discomfort. At night, she wakes up every couple of hours, and as a result I've gotten very little sleep. And when I do sleep, I'm continuing to have nightmares about trees falling, and now about being lost in the woods. I'm just so exhausted.

MATT: That sounds like so much for you.

CLAIRE: I've tried to not let my sister see this, but there are times when I just can't fight back the tears. The amount of loss . . . and the emotional pain I'm feeling. I don't mean to be selfish, and I know that I said I'm an optimistic person, but where's the justice in this?

MATT: It doesn't sound selfish to me, Claire; it just seems like there's so much going on with you right now.

CLAIRE: I was hoping that I was going to be able to have my sister as a source of support for me, but this has not been the case. Not at all. Also, I know we had talked about taking my sister's dog for a walk so I could exercise, but not only do I not have the energy or desire to do this, the dog only seems to want to stay in the backyard.

MATT: Claire, have you been able to find any sense of relief the past couple of days?

CLAIRE: No, not at all. I don't have much of an appetite, and even when I try to distract myself by reading, I simply can't stay focused. Even when I'm here now trying to look through the debris, I feel a pull to get back to my sister within the next two hours. I want to do all I can to help her, but in all honesty, who's going to help me?

MATT: It seems that you've been working very hard to take care of your sister, and it's pretty remarkable that you've been trying to take care of yourself on top of that. That speaks volumes to me about the type of person you are, but you need some help.

CLAIRE: I don't like to admit it, but I do.

MATT: Is it okay if we start with you?

CLAIRE: I think my sister needs help more.

MATT, *five-second pause*: But is it okay if we start with you?

CLAIRE, *five-second pause*: Okay.

MATT: I'm concerned that you're not able to get the support from your sister right now. I'm also concerned about the nightmares you're having, and your lack of eating and exercising. You need some time to take care of yourself, and you need some support and help doing this. There are free local counseling services that have been set up to assist those who are experiencing emotional difficulties as a result of the storms. It seems like you could benefit from these services.

CLAIRE: I suppose I could. I'm feeling really overwhelmed right now. But what about my sister?

MATT: There are also free medical services, including home health nursing, being offered. This might benefit your sister, as well as you.

CLAIRE: Really!? Just hearing that, Matt, makes me feel like a tremendous weight has been lifted from my shoulders.

MATT: I'm glad to hear that, Claire. If you'd like, we can make the call to them together now?

CLAIRE: That sounds good to me. Let's do that.

Scenario 2 Follow-Up Summary

This is a much different encounter than the first follow-up scenario. Claire is clearly not doing well. She is experiencing a lack of social support now that her sister is hurt, and she is overwhelmed. She is not sleeping well and continues to have nightmares. Her eating is poor and she's expressing signs of sadness, poor concentration, and anhedonia, all signs of depression. She needs help.

Matt used reflective listening techniques to provide support and encouragement to Claire. He also was able to offer and then facilitate access to the next level of care. This was fortunate but not always available. However, within this scenario, it highlights the need to assist in making a plan and having a sense of knowing what direction to go.

Mistakes to Avoid

In this scenario, Claire is overwhelmed, and it is apparent that she could use additional help. Claire is a compassionate, caring person who is focused on her sister. Matt is aware of this, acknowledges it, but then attempts to have Claire focus on herself. Consider, instead, the following exchange:

CLAIRE: I've tried to not let my sister see this, but there are times when I just can't fight back the tears. The amount of loss, and the emotional pain I'm feeling. I don't mean to be selfish, and I know that I said I'm an optimistic person, but where's the justice in this?

MATT: This doesn't sound like much justice at all. You've been trying to do too much. Maybe it's time to be a bit selfish?

CLAIRE: I'm sorry, but I just can't be that way. Not now.

MATT: What other options do you have? At this time, you need to take care of yourself.

Matt underestimates the connection Claire apparently has with her sister. Asking her to be selfish, though well intentioned, is premature and too direct. It's reasonable to suggest to someone to take care of herself before taking care of someone else, but the timing of this exchange is likely too abrupt.

Scenario 3 Follow-Up

In the preceding follow-up exchange, it was suggested that Claire would benefit from seeking the next level of care more immediately with a counselor. However, let's see what could occur if Claire were doing even more poorly. Consider the following exchange:

MATT: Hi, Claire!

CLAIRE, *quietly and with very little inflection in her voice*: Hello, Matt.

MATT: How are you doing?

CLAIRE: I'm sorry. What?

MATT: How are you doing?

CLAIRE: I'm not sure it's worth it.

MATT: Not worth it. What's not worth it?

CLAIRE: Anything.

Pause, 15 seconds of silence.

Anything at all!

Another 10-second pause.

When you left the other day, I looked and looked for something . . . anything, but I found nothing . . . nothing. I feel so hurt and so lost . . . I have nothing.

MATT: Claire, I'm so sorry that you haven't found anything of material relevance yet.

CLAIRE: It's not just that.

MATT: Not just that . . . there's more?

CLAIRE: There is just so much more.

MATT: It seems that you're overwhelmed with so much happening. Where would you like to begin?

CLAIRE: Where to begin . . . (*pause for 10 seconds*) where to begin?

Fifteen-second pause.

MATT, *sensing she needs additional direction*: Let me ask it this way. What's been the worst part of all of this for you so far?

CLAIRE: I've lost the things that remind me of Jim and Marissa. And I don't want to rebuild the house. I want it all to go away.

MATT: Claire, I'm concerned when I hear you say you want it all to go away. What do you mean?

CLAIRE: I want the pain to go away. I don't want to hurt this way anymore. I want to be with Jim.

MATT: You want to be with Jim?

CLAIRE: Jim suffered, and I watched him suffer, but then it was over for him, and I actually felt some relief. I can't stop thinking of wanting that relief.

MATT: Claire, when you say "wanting that relief," are you saying that you are thinking about hurting or killing yourself?

CLAIRE, *15-second pause, through tears*: I just don't want to live anymore.

MATT: Are you sure that you don't want to live anymore, or is it that you just don't want to have things continue the way they are right now?

CLAIRE: I just don't see it getting any better.

MATT: I believe it will get better . . . it will. Time will help, but you really need to give it time.

CLAIRE: Time might help, but then again, it might not! Right now, I don't see it getting any better. I'm exhausted, and I want the pain to stop.

MATT: I understand that you're feeling this way. A lot of people who experience these thoughts have them for about 24 to 72 hours.

CLAIRE: Well, I'm certainly feeling this way right now.

MATT: It's clear that you're hurting, Claire. Can you tell me where you hurt?

CLAIRE: I hurt all over. I hurt in places you can't imagine. And I've been thinking for the past day and a half how to make it end.

MATT: Thinking about how to make it end . . . so you have a plan?

CLAIRE: As you know, I've been staying with my sister, but she didn't tell me that when she went to check on the water in her basement, she slipped on the steps and fell, bruising her hip badly and twisting her ankle. I've needed to wait on her; she's in a lot of discomfort, and I'm just exhausted. She's been prescribed pain medication, and since yesterday I started looking online about how to do it. I've been thinking more and more about what it would be like to take her medication . . . a lot of it, with enough alcohol . . . and then be done with it.

MATT: Claire, I'm so sorry that you're feeling this way, but I'm glad you trusted me enough to share this with me. Is this your only plan?

CLAIRE, *pause for 10 seconds*: Yes.

MATT: I want to help you.

CLAIRE: How can you help me? You can't make this go away?

MATT: You're right, Claire, I can't. But I want to get you to people who can help. You have not been sleeping, eating, exercising, or finding any relief. You're emotionally overwhelmed, exhausted, and depressed. As a result, you're describing feeling excruciating pain. You need to get some relief from this pain. And this can be done! I know it might sound like a lot, but it can be done.

CLAIRE: I'm just not sure.

MATT: Have you ever attempted suicide?

CLAIRE: I thought about it after Jim died.

MATT: What stopped you from trying?

CLAIRE: I'm just not sure, but probably because I wasn't sure how to do it.

MATT: But now you have a plan and a way to do it.

CLAIRE: Yup!

MATT: Claire, you have experienced a tremendous loss now and other equally tremendous losses in your past; yet, you were able to get through them. How were you able to do this?

CLAIRE: I don't know. I was younger then, and my sister was there to help me.

MATT: And once she's better, she can be there again to help you. And what would it be like for her if you're not there?

CLAIRE: I don't know. It just feels like so much.

MATT: And what about your daughter, son-in-law, and granddaughter? They're expecting you soon.

CLAIRE: I know. But I just want to be left alone.

MATT: Claire, I'm not going to be able to leave you alone.

CLAIRE: So what do you want me to do?

MATT: I want you to come with me.

CLAIRE: Come with you? Where?

MATT: I want to find one of the EMTs who can take you to the hospital, so you can talk with people there who can help you.

CLAIRE, *15-second pause*: You're going to insist on this, aren't you?

MATT: I care, Claire.

CLAIRE: Will you stay with me?

MATT: Of course. I'm sure they will let me ride along, but if not, I will meet you at the hospital.

Scenario 3 Follow-Up Summary

Claire is clearly in despair and is demonstrating dysfunction. Fortunately, she confides this to Matt but is not particularly subtle in her description. This is a PFA provider's worst-case scenario. Matt responds, however, by establishing very directly that Claire has suicidal ideation, in addition to a plan. It is generally considered that being direct with someone who is suicidal is better than trying to evade or even bypass the topic. Matt also establishes that this is Claire's only current plan and that she has thought about it in the past. Matt attempts to keep Claire future oriented (i.e., seeing her daughter and granddaughter) and to provide her with the realization that although she may have had the thoughts previously, she did not act on them. Matt then establishes that he is not going to leave Claire alone. In this scenario, and likely based on the trust and rapport they established, she acquiesces and even asks him to stay. However, if she objected, and let's say abruptly left and drove away, Matt would have had to call for other assistance, possibly police, paramedics, or a supervisory disaster relief worker.

Mistakes to Avoid

Being with someone who is actively suicidal is challenging. And even though this is a rare occurrence when doing PFA, it is worth noting and reviewing. Having the person remain alive is the goal, *not* fixing all of their problems, so if that is achieved, you are successful.

All persons who are at risk for suicide need help. Moreover, it is always better to overreact, in terms of actions you take, than to fail to take action. It also is much better to have someone angry with you or feel embarrassed than it is to find him or her dead. However, there are some tactics you should avoid when assessing someone who is potentially suicidal. For example, do not minimize his or her concerns (e.g., this is not worth killing yourself over, it's not so bad, or others have it much worse), do not make light of the threat (e.g., you don't really want to kill yourself), and do not tell him or her you know how he or she feels, or, as noted above, evoke God (this was God's will). Consider, for example, the following exchange:

MATT: Claire, when you say "wanting that relief," are you saying that you are thinking about hurting or killing yourself?

CLAIRE, *15-second pause, through tears*: I just don't want to live anymore.

MATT: You don't want to kill yourself . . .

CLAIRE: I just don't see it getting any better.

MATT: Losing your home and taking care of your sister are just not worth killing yourself over. There's nothing you could do about these things.

CLAIRE: I feel that I've lost so much.

MATT: In this instance, you lost a home . . . a home. This can be replaced, and your sister will get better. In reality, Claire, it's just not that bad. Others lost much more.

CLAIRE: I know that, but . . .

MATT: Maybe this current pain is something you need to experience at this time in your life. Although it isn't pleasant, have you thought of that?

As you can see, Matt is minimizing Claire's concerns and is discounting her suicidal threat. The impact of doing this might be profound. Fortunately, proper training in PFA makes this type of exchange a rare occurrence.

KEY POINT SUMMARY

The disposition phase of the RAPID PFA model is critically important as it is most likely the end of the intervention, other than perhaps follow-up. It is hoped that this phase serves as a bit of a crescendo where the person's acute state of distress or dysfunction has been mitigated. Furthermore, you have been successful in providing some degree of reassurance and plant a realistic seed of hope for a better tomorrow.

Possible steps in disposition:

1. Summarize the main points of the interaction you've just had.
2. Ask the person how they are feeling right now.
3. Make a plan for next steps: "Where do we go from here?"
4. Delineate specific steps necessary.
5. Tactically facilitate access to another level of care, if necessary.
6. Otherwise, make plans for follow-up.
7. Try to offer some realistic words of hope or encouragement.

References

American Psychiatric Association. (1954). *Psychological first aid in community disasters*. Washington, DC: American Psychiatric Association.

McCabe, O. L., Everly, G. S., Jr., Brown, L. M., Wendelboe, A. M., Abd Hamid, N. H., Tallchief, V. L., & Links, J. M. (2014). Psychological first aid: A consensus-derived, empirically supported, competency-based training model. *American Journal of Public Health, 104*, 621–628. http://dx.doi .org/10.2105/AJPH.2013.301219.

Raphael, B. (1986). *When disaster strikes: How individuals and communities cope with catastrophe*. New York, NY: Basic Books.

PSYCHOLOGICAL FIRST AID

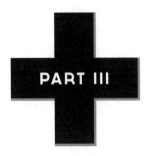

FURTHER CONSIDERATIONS

In this third and final part of the book, we extend our discussion of psychological first aid (PFA) into important application areas. When it comes to disaster and even well-circumscribed adversity, children represent an extraordinarily vulnerable population. Given the relative lack of mental health practitioners who specialize in children and their unique developmental and situational vulnerabilities, PFA may represent an important means of providing at least initial psychological support that might lessen the severity and long-term impact of adversity. In chapter 10, we consider how the RAPID PFA model might be adapted to work with children.

Sensitivity to culturally defined or culturally influenced aspects of the human experience is critical when providing PFA as well. In chapter 11, we raise awareness of this important dynamic and suggest how it might influence provider effectiveness. And in chapter 12 we describe community-based PFA. As observed by the United Nations and others, there is a critical shortage of psychological support services in many communities. The increase in disasters and community violence coupled with growing numbers of marginalized and underserved persons argues for a new approach to the provision of psychological support at the community level. We believe community PFA can serve to effectively expand community surge capacity as well as expand the total fabric of mental health care.

Finally, the provision of psychological support in disaster and other types of adversity is not without a cost. Self-care not only fosters resilience, but we believe it is necessary to maintain one's overall effectiveness in the provision of PFA. We offer guidance for self-care in chapter 13.

TEN | RAPID PFA Considerations with Children

THE FOCUS OF THIS TEXT has been on how to provide the Johns Hopkins RAPID PFA model with adults. However, we realize what was missing from the first edition are some suggestions of how RAPID PFA might be modified to apply to children. This chapter is not meant to provide an exhaustive review of the types of trauma children might experience or to reiterate information that has already been covered in previous chapters in regards to foundational information associated with the five RAPID phases. Instead, the purpose is to provide suggestions for PFA providers on how they might adapt each of the five RAPID PFA phases when working with children. Where appropriate, we will offer suggestions on how these adaptations might currently be impacted by COVID-19.

Background Information

Traumatic events are thought to impact as many as 80% of children worldwide (Sharma-Patel et al., 2011). Data have also shown, however, that fortunately most children, similar to adults, exhibit resilience in the aftermath of critical incidents (particularly single-incident exposure and particularly if they have access to caring adults who assist them in integrating this experience into their worldview) (Briere & Scott, 2006; Maikoetter, 2011; US Department of Health and Human Services, 2013). However, some children exposed to critical incidents experience a disruption in psychological equilibrium or balance because their coping mechanisms have failed, and this can result in distress and functional impairment (Caplan, 1964).

Researchers have previously noted that parents, teachers, and even mental health professionals may underestimate the duration and intensity of accompanying stress reactions that occur in children to traumatic events (Amaya-Jackson, 2000; Schreier et al., 2005; Webb, 2006). Moreover, as noted by Kar (2009), "Depending upon the developmental stage, level of cognitive and emotional maturity, and limited coping strategies, the psychological reactions in children are expected to be different from those in adults" (p. 5). The burgeoning work in the past several decades on the psychological impact of traumatic events on children continues to explore and address these salient issues.

A unique consideration in providing PFA with children, compared to working with adults, is the need to seek parental or guardian permission, except under emergent conditions (e.g., if the child is a danger to self or others). Pynoos and Nader (1988) noted more than 30 years ago that a critical first step for providing successful on-site PFA with children is "establishing a direct, open and mutually supportive relationship with the adult authorities in charge" (p. 456). Therefore, sound practice for a PFA provider is to establish a connection with a parent or guardian before speaking with a child or adolescent to explain the purpose of the encounter and the provider's role. However, if an interventionist speaks to a child in distress when no adult is present, the PFA provider should locate a parent or caregiver as soon as possible to let them know about what transpired (National Child Traumatic Stress Network, 2006). With these general background caveats in mind, we can offer suggestions on how each of the RAPID PFA stages might be modified to work with children.

Rapport and Reflective Listening

Regardless of the child's age, it is important for PFA providers to be emotionally present and work to establish a safe environment that demonstrates availability, willingness to listen, and supportiveness (Field, Wehrman, & Yoo, 2017). This is predicated on PFA providers being flexible in their approach, emitting calmness and composure (both verbally and nonverbally), and recognizing that the basic premise of effective PFA is assisting others in finding words or behaviors to help them communicate. It often begins tactically by fostering stabilization, such as finding a quiet place to talk, and then asking the child if they are physically hurting, need anything to eat or drink, or would like something to enhance comfort (e.g., favorite toy, stuffed animal, or blanket). It is often helpful in establishing safety and trust for the PFA provider, if appropriate and if the child is comfortable, to move closer to eye level with the child; this might involve sitting on the floor.

Over the past decade, considerable efforts have been made to utilize advances in technology to facilitate telehealth, or videoconferencing-based practice (Grady et al., 2011). These remote efforts have flourished since the outbreak of COVID-19, due to social distancing, limited access to care, and burgeoning need, even though there is a paucity of current empirical evidence supporting its use with children and adolescents (Ros-DeMarize, Chung, & Stewart, 2021). While the RAPID PFA model was intended to be delivered in person, as noted in chapter 2, given the current restrictions regarding in-person meetings, it might be necessary, if other options are unavailable, to provide the model remotely. If this occurs, obvious adjustments to establishing rapport will be required (e.g., offering something to drink or enhancing comfort by offering a toy); however, the foundations of emitting calmness and composure clearly remain.

Once a sense of safety and rapport is established, PFA providers should state directly to the child that they know about the critical incident and that the purpose of their time together is to help reduce the child's worries and gain some strength by talking or maybe even playing (Webb, 2006). It is important for the PFA provider to use active listening and reflective statements while making it clear that he or she is willing to hear everything the child has to say (Pynoos & Nader, 1988). Similar to working with adults, this willingness provides a perception of control, along with helping to foster the relationship. For example, the PFA provider should allow the child to choose where they sit, or if they walk and talk, play and talk, or even draw and talk. Also, while the PFA provider should ask if the child wants to talk about what happened, if the choice is not to talk, the interventionist should not attempt to compel him or her to speak about it. The PFA provider may instead ask the child how their body feels, what they might be worried about, or even more generally what they *do* want to talk about (Field, Wehrman, & Yoo, 2017). If the child continues to choose not to talk, the PFA provider might escort the child back to where they met but ask about checking in a bit later or even establishing a "signal" that the child might use to let the provider know when they are ready to talk. It is also worth noting that if the child chooses to talk about what happened, it is prudent to be cautious about not having them tell the story repeatedly, particularly to other people, to avoid retraumatization (Briere & Scott, 2006).

Assessment

As noted in chapter 6, assessment relies on the physical and psychological information provided by the person in distress and is used by the interventionist to determine the need for PFA. The symptoms of psychological trauma in children are heterogeneous and can also vary depending on the child's age and developmental stage. While a thorough review of childhood developmental stages and factors affecting resilience are beyond the scope of this chapter, we offer the following general descriptions of age groups and accompanying emotional reactions to critical incidents that PFA providers might encounter.

Preschool-aged children (ages five years and younger) exposed to traumatic events will often model the reactions of adults around them. Therefore, adults maintaining a calm demeanor, while admittedly challenging during and often after critical incidents, can help to mitigate some of the typically exhibited behaviors in preschool children, such as frequent crying, agitation, hyperarousal, separation anxiety (e.g., not being able to fall asleep without a caregiver with them), difficulty using words to describe what they are experiencing, regression to earlier developmental stages (e.g., bed-wetting, thumb-sucking, toys they play with), and refusal to follow directions (Field, Wehrman, & Yoo, 2017; Markese, 2011; US Department of Health and Human Services, 2019). Possibly predicated in part by the reactions of adults, qualitative data from 67 New York City parents of 104 children (with an average age of 4.4 years) living in close proximity to Ground Zero on the day of the September 11 attacks reported that many of the children unexpectedly, and also possibly due to being withdrawn or in shock, reacted in a calm and cooperative manner by listening to directions (such as wearing masks), quietly playing by themselves, and in some instances falling asleep (Klein et al., 2009).

In the aftermath of traumatic exposure, children between the ages of 6 and 11 years might experience difficulties in school (e.g., poor attention, poor concentration, and disruptive behavior), isolation from friends and family, and sleep disturbances (including refusing to go to bed, difficulty falling asleep, and nightmares) (American Psychological Association, 2008; US Department of Health and Human Services, 2019). They may also use play, artwork, or storytelling to recreate the event; complain of physical problems that are uncommon for them (e.g., headaches, stomachaches); develop superstitious behaviors, unfounded fears, or "magical thinking" (e.g., that they somehow caused the event); express feeling guilty if they thought they were somehow culpable for the event; and lose interest and desire to participate in enjoyable activities (US Department of Health and Human Services, 2019).

Adolescents between the ages of 12 and 17 years who have been exposed to critical incidents are similar to younger children in that they might demonstrate concentration, academic, and behavioral problems at school. They might also exhibit sleep problems, including nightmares and insomnia, as well as somatic complaints. In addition, because adolescent development involves identity formation (Schwartz et al., 2013), it is possible that the effects of traumatic events can influence decision making that can lead to acting out or thrill-seeking behaviors, such as alcohol, drug or tobacco use, or sexual promiscuity. Issues of guilt for not preventing deaths or injuries might happen, as well as thoughts of revenge (US Department of Health and Human Services, 2019). In more extreme cases of adolescents who experienced adverse life events and report trauma symptoms (e.g., PTSD and depression), self-injurious behaviors with suicide intent might occur (Zetterqvist, Lundh, & Svedin, 2013).

Psychological Triage/Prioritization

Psychological triage or prioritization is used to determine the order in which the interventionist responds to the signs, symptoms, and specific needs of those in distress. A general consideration in prioritizing crisis reactions with children includes recognizing differences between externalizing and internalizing behaviors. Externalizing behaviors such as anger, frustration, negative attitude, verbal outbursts, physical aggression, power struggles with teachers and adults, and substance use are more outwardly expressive, whereas internalizing behaviors consist, for example, of sadness, loneliness, guilt, crying, and self-injurious behavior (Field, Wehrman, & Yoo, 2017; Kranzler et al., 2016; van der Kolk, 2003). Children who demonstrate externalizing behaviors, which are thought to be mediated by anger, are more likely to get noticed at home and at school than are those with more internalizing behaviors, which are thought to be mediated by depression (Asgeirsdottir et al., 2011). In a systematic review of the impact of social isolation and loneliness on children and adolescents in the context of COVID-19 (i.e., internalizing behaviors), Loades et al. (2020) reported that loneliness was most strongly associated with depression and that enforced isolation (i.e., quarantine) led to five times the need for mental health services and increased levels of posttraumatic stress. Also, self-injurious behavior, which it was noted to look for in the assessment phase, is an internalized action that can often go unnoticed but is clearly quite severe and warrants an urgent prioritized response, as do more aberrant external behaviors, such as substance use.

Intervention

Chapter 8 provided a list of specific intervention tactics for PFA providers to consider, and as noted in the introduction to this chapter, those are not repeated here. We do, however, offer some examples of how some of these tactics might be implemented or amended for working with children. For example, as with adults, critical elements for helping to mitigate distress in children are social support and, as noted in the rapport section, enhancing the perception of control. In addition to offering specific choices to enhance perception of control, another way to empower a child is through explanatory guidance. For instance, when children experience physical and emotional reactions in themselves, or observe them in others, they can become panicked, not only over what is occurring but also over their thoughts and feelings. In these situations, it is helpful to offer explanatory guidance in age-appropriate terms (such as metaphors or animal stories) about how the body works when stressed or frightened (Gaffney, 2006). This type of normalizing can be very powerful for children (as it is with adults) since it lets them know that others are likely experiencing similar distress responses. In response to the current COVID-19 outbreak and its impact on structure, normalcy, and grief, Sullivan (2021) suggests that the use of storytelling can be used to increase communication, identify emotions, reduce stress, and foster resilience. Also, children who might be expressing magical thinking, such that they were involved in some way in causing the incident, will benefit from assistance in understanding and normalizing the true cause of the event so they do not become preoccupied with guilt.

Another empowering strategy, and one also consistent when working with adults, is to ask children to describe what they have done in the past to help them get through challenging times. Depending on the child's age, the interventionist can modify the questions by asking, for example, "What do you do to feel better when you are sad, upset, or lonely? How does it work? What do you think can make it work even better? What else can you think of to help you?" Some younger, more verbal children with vivid imaginations may offer creative, if not fantasy-laden, solutions to their stressful difficulties (Gaffney, 2006). For some children who struggle with these questions, and even for those who do not, Gaffney (2006) also notes that it might be helpful to suggest to younger children that they find a special, safe place that they can fill with their favorite things and then use as needed for time alone to think, reflect, or relax—what she refers to as "finding sanctuary" (p. 1011).

For younger, less verbal children, the use of drawing or play, which are often considered symbolic language, may be used to help foster expression and healing by helping to clarify information, including misinformation, and to create or provide meaning to the critical incident (Eaton, Doherty, & Widrick, 2007; Webb, 2006). An example of this type of cognitive reframing, or clarifying misinformation, tactic with more verbal children is for the PFA provider to acknowledge the child's bravery (e.g., going to school, going outside, being alone, or even in the moment by talking with him or her).

For older children and adolescents, other intervention approaches that are comparable to working with adults might be used, such as suggesting books to read (e.g., *The PTSD Survival Guide for Teens: Strategies to Overcome Trauma, Build Resilience, and Take Back Your Life* by Sheela Raja and Jaya Raja Ashrafi, 2018), journaling, music, relaxation techniques (e.g., diaphragmatic breathing, meditation, yoga, progressive relaxation), and exercise (de Arellano et al., 2005; Everly & Lating, 2019). However, if suspected drug or alcohol use is occurring, it is important to directly ask about it (refer to chapter 3 on assessment strategies) and to describe to children that alcohol is an unwanted chemical that is being released into the brain that is interfering with the stress chemicals that are concurrently being released in an attempt to keep them alert, focused, and functioning. A PFA provider may then note that they do not need any other chemicals right now in their brains. Another consideration, and offered in chapters 3 and 8, is to advise children and adolescents about the dangers of consuming caffeinated energy drinks or using tobacco, including electronic nicotine delivery systems (e.g., e-cigarettes or vapes).

Lastly, and as noted in chapter 9, potential suicidal or self-harm risk is by far the most daunting and challenging aspect of doing PFA work. Fortunately, it is an exceedingly rare occurrence before puberty (Shaffer et al., 2001) and a rare occurrence in general when providing PFA. However, part of effective crisis management is to be prepared for the worst-case scenario (see Substance Abuse Mental Health Services Administration [2009] for guidelines on interacting with persons in suicide crisis). So, if faced with a self-injurious behavior possibility when working with an older child or adolescent, the interventionist should speak in a calm, nonaccusatory manner; dispute irrational thinking (e.g., that the child will feel like this forever); and most importantly, err on the side of safety and caution by informing parents and facilitating immediate access to the next level of care (e.g., emergency room, pediatrician), as in the scenario with Claire in chapter 9.

Disposition

After formulating a plan and then implementing it with a child, the interventionist needs to consider the disposition and potential follow-up, or next steps. While providing the PFA, this often entails summarizing what has been discussed, asking how the child is currently feeling, talking about action plans, and providing words of gratitude for the child's willingness and comfort in talking. If, as indicated above, next level of care is required immediately, these specific arrangements need to be made swiftly and tactfully. Otherwise, within a day or two of the RAPID PFA, follow-up with the child's parent and child is expected and good practice. In most cases this follow-up consists of assessing how the child is doing, continuing to normalize reactions, and answering questions. In some instances, parents may seek referrals for community resources, including agencies that provide basic needs (e.g., food, clothing, shelter), financial resources, health care referrals (e.g., therapists who do play therapy or trauma-focused therapy), or faith-based referrals.

KEY POINT SUMMARY

1. The core features of the Johns Hopkins RAPID PFA model can be adapted and applied to children.

2. A unique consideration in providing RAPID PFA with children is the need to seek parental or guardian permission, except under emergent conditions.

3. Rapport in working with children is established by the interventionist being calm and composed, meeting basic needs, being open to listening, providing choices, and being flexible in helping children tell their stories. Adjustments, as needed, can be made during the COVID-19 pandemic.

4. Assessment with children is facilitated by being aware of some of the typical responses they might emit depending on their age and developmental level.

5. Psychological triage/prioritization can be enhanced when working with children by recognizing the difference and impact of internalizing and externalizing behaviors.

6. Intervention techniques with children can include normalizing distress responses using age-appropriate terms, empowering them, and using cognitive reframing to help clarify information and provide meaning. For older children and adolescents, stress management techniques such as journaling, relaxation, and exercise can be offered.

7. Disposition with children entails summarizing main points, offering words of gratitude and hope, and if required under emergency situations (e.g., potential harm), taking the steps required for access

to the next level of care. Follow-up plans with the child and parents are then arranged.

References

Amaya-Jackson, L. (2000). Posttraumatic stress disorder in children and adolescents. In B. Sadock & V. Sadock (Eds.), *Kaplan and Sadock's comprehensive textbook of psychiatry* (7th ed., pp. 63–69). Philadelphia, PA: Lippincott Williams and Wilkins.

American Psychological Association. (2008). *Children and trauma: Update for mental health professionals.* APA Presidential Task Force on Posttraumatic Stress Disorder and Trauma in Children and Adolescents. Washington, DC. Government Relations Office.

Asgeirsdottir, B. B., Sigfusdottir, I. D., Gudjonsson, G. H., & Sigurdsson, J. F. (2011). Association between sexual abuse and family conflict/violence, self-injurious behavior, and substance use: The mediating role of depressed mood and anger. *Child Abuse & Neglect, 35,* 210–219. http://dx.doi .org/10.1016/j.chiabu.2010.12.003.

Briere, J., & Scott, C. (2006). *Principles of trauma therapy: A guide to symptoms, evaluation, and treatment.* Thousand Oaks, CA: Sage.

Caplan, G. (1964). *Principles of preventive psychiatry.* New York, NY: Basic Books.

de Arellano, M. A., Waldrop, A. E., Deblinger, E., Cohen, J. A., Danielson, C. K., & Mannarino, A. R. (2005). Community outreach program for child victims of traumatic events: A community-based project for underserved populations. *Behavior Modification, 29,* 130–155. http://dx.doi.org/10.1177 /0145445504270878.

Eaton, L. G., Doherty, K. L. & Widrick, R. M. (2007). A review of research and methods used to establish art therapy as an effective treatment method for traumatized children. *The Arts in Psychotherapy, 34,* 256–262. http://dx .doi.org/10.1016/j.aip.2007.03.001.

Everly, G. S., Jr., & Lating, J. M. (2019). *A clinical guide to the treatment of the human stress response* (4th ed.). New York, NY: Springer Nature.

Field, J. E., Wehrman, J. D., & Yoo, M. S. (2017). Helping the weeping, worried, and willful: Psychological first aid for primary and secondary students. *Journal of Asia Pacific Counseling, 7,* 169–180. http://dx.doi.org/10.18401/2017 .2.4.

Gaffney, D. A. (2006). The aftermath of disaster: Children in crisis. *Journal of Clinical Psychology: In Session, 62,* 1001–1016. http://dx.doi.org/10.1002/jclp.20285.

Grady, B., Myers, K. M., Nelson, E-L., Belz, N., Bennett, L., Carnahan, L., . . . Voyles, D. (2011). Evidence-based practice for telemental health. *Telemedicine and e-Health, 17.* http://dx.doi.org/10.1089/tmj.2010.0158.

Kar, N. (2009). Psychological impact of disasters on children: Review of assessment and interventions. *World Journal of Pediatrics, 5,* 5–11. http://dx.doi.org/10.1007/s12519-009-0001-x.

Klein, T. P., Devoe, E. R., Miranda-Julian, C., & Linas, K. (2009). Young children's responses to September 11th: The New York City experience. *Infant Mental Health Journal, 30,* 1–22. http://dx.doi.org/10.1002/imhj.20200.

Kranzler, A., Fehling, K. B., Anestis, M. D., & Selby, E. A. (2016). Emotional dysregulation, internalizing symptoms, and self-injurious and suicidal behavior: Structural equation modeling analysis. *Death Studies, 40,* 358–366. http://dx.doi.org/10.1080/07481187.2016.1145156.

Loades, M. E., Chatburn, E., Higson-Sweeney, N., Reynolds, S., Shafran, R., Brigden, A., . . . Crawley, E. (2020). Rapid systematic review: The impact of social isolation and loneliness on the mental health of children and adolescents in the context of COVID-19. *Journal of the American Academy of Child & Adolescent Psychiatry, 59,* 1218-1239e3. http://dx.doi.org/10.1016/j.jaac.2020.05.009.

Maikoetter, M. (2011). From intuition to science: Re-ED and trauma informed care. *Reclaiming Children and Youth, 19,* 18–22.

Markese, S. (2011). Dyadic trauma in infancy and early childhood: Review of the literature. *Journal of Infant, Child, and Adolescent Psychotherapy, 10,* 341–378. http://dx.doi.org/10.1080/15289168.2011.600214.

National Child Traumatic Stress Network (2006). *Psychological first aid: Field operations guide* (2nd ed.). Retrieved March 23, 2021, from http://www.nctsn.org/resources/psychological-first-aid-pfa-field-operations-guide-2nd-edition.

Pynoos, R. S., & Nader, K. (1988). Psychological first aid and treatment approach to children exposed to community violence: Research implications. *Journal of Traumatic Stress, 1,* 445–473. http://dx.doi.org/10.1002/jts.2490010406.

Raja, S., & Ashrafi, J. R. (2018). *The PTSD survival guide for teens: Strategies to overcome trauma, build resilience, and take back your life.* Oakland, CA: New Harbinger Publications.

Ros-DeMarize, R., Chung, P., & Stewart, R. (2021). Pediatric behavioral telehealth in the age of COVID-19: Brief evidence and practice considerations. *Current Problems in Pediatric and Adolescent Health Care, 51*, 100949. http://dx.doi.org/10.1016/j.cppeds.2021.100949.

Schreier, H., Ladakakos, C., Morabito, D., Chapman, L., & Knudson, M. M. (2005). Posttraumatic stress symptoms in children after mild to moderate pediatric trauma: A longitudinal examination of symptom prevalence, correlates, and parent-child symptom reporting. *Journal of Trauma, Injury, Infection, and Critical Care, 58*, 353–363. http://dx.doi.org/10.1097/01.TA .0000152537.15672.B7.

Schwartz, S. J., Zamboanga, B. L., Luyckx, K., Meca, A., & Ritchie, R. A. (2013). Identity in emerging adulthood: Reviewing the field and looking forward. *Emerging Adulthood, 1*, 96–113. http://dx.doi.org/10.1177/2167696813479781.

Shaffer, D., Pfeffer, C. R., and the Workgroup on Quality Issues (2001). Practice parameter for the assessment and treatment of children and adolescents with suicidal behavior. *Journal of the American Academy of Child & Adolescent Psychiatry, 40*, 24S–51S. http://dx.doi.org/10.1097/00004583 -200107001-00003.

Sharma-Patel, K., Filton, B., Brown, E., Zlotnik, D., Campbell, C., & Yeldin, J. (2011). Pediatric posttraumatic stress disorder. In D. McKay & E. A. Storch (Eds.), *Handbook of child and adolescent anxiety disorders* (pp. 303–322). New York, NY: Springer.

Substance Abuse and Mental Health Services Administration (2009). *Practice guidelines: Core elements for responding to mental health crises.* HHS Publication No. SMA-09-4427. Rockville, MD: Center for Mental Health Services.

Sullivan, M. A. (2021). The use of storytelling with grief reactions in children during the COVID-19 pandemic. *Journal of Psychosocial Nursing and Mental Health Services, 59*, 13–15. http://dx.doi.org/10.3928/02793695-20201015-02.

US Department of Health and Human Services, National Institutes of Health, National Institute of Mental Health. (2013). *Helping children and adolescents cope with violence and disasters: For parents of children exposed to violence or disaster, what parents can do* (NIH Publication No. 13-3518). Bethesda, MD: Government Printing Office.

US Department of Health and Human Services, National Institutes of Health, National Institute of Mental Health. (2019). *Helping children and adolescents cope with disasters and other traumatic events: What parents, rescue workers, and the community can do* (NIH Publication No. 19-MH-8066). Bethesda, MD: Government Printing Office.

van der Kolk, B. A. (2003). The neurobiology of childhood trauma and abuse. *Child and Adolescent Psychiatric Clinics of North America, 12,* 293–317. http://dx.doi.org/10.1016/S1056-4993(03)00003-8.

Webb, N. B. (2006). Crisis intervention play therapy to help traumatized children. In L. Carey (Ed.), *Expressive and creative arts methods for trauma survivors* (pp. 39–56). London and Philadelphia: Jessica Kingsley Publishers.

Zetterqvist, M., Lundh, L.-G., & Svedin, C. G. (2013). A comparison of adolescents engaging in self-injurious behaviors with and without suicidal intent: Self-reported experiences of adverse life events and trauma symptoms. *Journal of Youth and Adolescence, 42,* 1257–1272. http://dx.doi.org/10.1007/s10964-012-9872-6.

ELEVEN | Cultural Awareness and Psychological First Aid

AS NOTED IN CHAPTER 4, natural disasters and human-made disasters are becoming ubiquitous. Aligned with these increased occurrences, including the coronavirus (COVID-19) pandemic, are the proliferation and accessibility of the global media, including social media, which has allowed for virtually immediate access and firsthand accounts of traumatic events anywhere in the world. This new globalism has in many respects made the world "smaller" by bringing increased information regarding exposure, often including graphic depictions of human suffering, from remote areas of the world to our attention. Providing faces to human suffering has not only led to increased sympathy for others in the aftermath of traumatic events but has also fostered interest, investment, and appreciation of differences among varied cultures.

The purpose of this text is to provide a step-by-step model to assess and help mitigate the emotional consequences of those exposed to critical incidents, with an emphasis on assessing each person's story and responses from his or her perspective. What we realized was missing, however, from the first edition was a description of how culture serves as a medium through which individuals shape, view, perceive, and respond to critical incidents. In fact, more than 25 years ago Weaver and Wodarski (1995) noted that "the importance of culture, which is a primary determining factor in a client's world view, is blatantly missing in most of the literature on crisis intervention" (p. 214). We want to continue to raise awareness and address this limitation. In chapter 4, we noted, for example, the disproportionate harm that COVID-19 has had on Black, Hispanic, and Asian people in the United States (Lopez, Hart, & Katz, 2021). We recognize, however, that the comprehensive coverage of the sociologic and applied implications of cultural awareness and competency, while extremely salient, are also extensive, complex, and beyond the scope of this text. Our intent in this chapter is not to be prescriptive or stereotypic but to instead provide cultural insights, considerations, and examples that might increase cultural awareness as a possible means to enhance proficiency when providing RAPID PFA.

Defining Relevant Terms and Concepts

It is generally agreed that the definition of culture entails a lens through which members of a group experience such shared constructs as knowledge, beliefs, morals, arts, and customs related to the world that are transmitted across time and generations (Kagawa-Singer et al., 2014; Triandis, 2007; Tylor, 1871). Culture is, therefore, considered to have material components, such as buildings and other tangible structures (e.g., artwork), as well as nonmaterial components, such as language, symbols, values, rituals, morals, and customs (Ogburn, 1966). During crises, individuals will often lean on their cultural beliefs for support, comfort, and guidance, so it is important that PFA providers recognize how cultural context influences how problems are identified, what solutions are considered, and what type of help or helpers are most appropriate to assist in assessing and mitigating signs of distress.

While it is advantageous for PFA providers to be versed in a variety of different cultures, it is clearly unrealistic for them to have working knowledge of all diverse groups. Another potentially relevant factor, and one that speaks to being cautious about stereotypically defining a culture, is that many people are exposed to or identify with more than one culture and are therefore considered multicultural. We recognize and appreciate that "differences among group members may be just as varied as the differences between members of one ethnocultural group and another. Thus, one should be mindful of such considerations when making sweeping generalizations about group characteristics or attributes" (Carswell & Carswell, 2008, p. 39).

We, therefore, support the need for PFA providers to enhance their cultural competency, which is considered to reflect one's own cultural awareness that then facilitates understanding, communicating, and interacting effectively with people across cultures and is based on openness, trust, equity, fairness, and social justice (Sue, Arredondo, & McDavis, 1992; Whaley & Davis, 2007). Within the past decade, West-Olatunji and Yoon (2013) have proposed a culture-centered model specific to "expeditiously respond to the needs of culturally diverse disaster-affected individuals" (p. 35). This crisis-based model is predicated on critical consciousness theory, which was developed by Brazilian educator Paulo Freire (1973) to help those who are disenfranchised to critically assess their social conditions and advocate for change (Watts, Diemer, & Voight, 2011). More specifically, West-Olatunji and Yoon (2013) propose general issues as well as individual factors to consider that may enhance cultural competency. Let us explore these factors.

Initial PFA Considerations

For those providing RAPID PFA, or for those providing training in PFA, it might be beneficial to include preincident preparation in cultural awareness, starting with an exploration of one's own worldviews, beliefs, and possible biases. It might then be helpful to facilitate training in mechanisms on how to acquire information related to the social and historical contexts of geographic areas where PFA providers may be referred (e.g., historical trauma, cultural differences between dominant and nondominant groups, and/or socially embedded stressors that occur in conjunction with the critical incident) (Halpern & Tramontin, 2007; Roysircar, 2004). One of the best ways to obtain this important information is consulting the literature before being deployed to unfamiliar communities, while another way is for providers to ask questions once they arrive on scene. Acquiring this information will likely not only enhance PFA providers' effectiveness in tactically providing the steps of the RAPID PFA model but will also help them better understand where and how to make next-level-of-care referrals if needed.

From an individual perspective, it is essential to be thoughtful and tempered when providing a RAPID PFA response. For example, it is important for providers not to allow the urgency of the critical incident to cloud, bias, or permit their own worldview to affect their willingness or ability to be open to hearing and learning about how impacted persons' perceptions of personal, cultural, and social history might influence their response. For instance, as noted by Pederson (1987), and particularly relevant for doing RAPID PFA, a Western view of problem solving usually consists of linear cause-and-effect thinking, whereas other cultures may have a more circular view, in which many other factors may be involved. Therefore, different cultures might have different definitions of success. For example, while some cultures might seek independence others might foster increased collaboration or codependency. Moreover, Pederson (1987) notes that it may be misguided at times to assume that individuals are the basic building blocks of all societies and therefore crisis intervention should be directed primarily toward individuals rather than groups, families, and organizations. Thus, for some cultures, and in some instances, it is worth considering the option of initially providing group-focused PFA rather than individual-focused PFA. As noted earlier, a randomized controlled trial conducted by Despeaux et al. (2019) demonstrated the efficacy of the group variant of RAPID PFA.

In addition to these general individual guidelines, we believe it is helpful to suggest how culture might influence some of the initial responses a PFA provider might encounter, including, as noted previously, the need to consider providing these services virtually during the COVID-19 pandemic. What makes these suggestions so potentially relevant is that the crux of RAPID PFA is predicated on quickly and effectively establishing a relationship. Therefore, any unintentional misunderstanding or violation of customs, rituals, or beliefs on the part of the RAPID PFA provider might prevent rapport from being established, or possibly worse, distance or offend the person or group the PFA provider is intending to help. Consider, for example, that one of the first identity variables a RAPID PFA provider should be prepared for and ask about is the person's preferred language. While it is clearly advantageous to have those of any cultural descent speak or use (e.g., in the case of sign language) their preferred language to help foster comfort and evoke emotional expression, the obvious limitation from a RAPID PFA perspective is the accessibility and availability of language-proficient providers or interpreters. If the preferred language cannot be used, yet the intervention continues in a nonpreferred and more questionably fluent language for the person receiving the intervention, the PFA provider should address this limitation and work to ensure that the information shared is being processed and understood. This can be facilitated by periodically checking on the pacing of the exchange, asking if the recipient has questions, or by having the recipient paraphrase received information to assess for accuracy and comprehension.

Another initial PFA cultural consideration is the location of the critical incident. In urban (city) areas, and depending on the scale of the incident, local authorities are typically responsible for disaster-related strategic plans and operations, such as providing supplies, shelters, and equipment to those in need (Barzinpour & Esmaeili, 2014). Often included in these plans are organizational policies and procedures for dealing with psychological trauma, including developing, training, and evaluating PFA (Forbes et al., 2011). Urban life is complex but has been noted to affect the production, consumption, and literal definition of culture (Turley, 2016). We are aware, however, of the heterogeneity of traumatic events, including that such natural disasters as tornados and floods frequently have a more devastating impact in rural areas. PFA providers, when responding to these areas, should be aware that many of these regions are thought to have their own distinct culture. Riding-Malon and Werth (2014) suggest that within rural communities there is the "presence of complex, interrelated networks with deep historical, social, familial, and political roots; strong family ties; avoiding conflict or discussing feelings; stoic attitudes toward life in general; and high involvement in religious activities in their communities" (p. 86). PFA providers should be aware of how these, and other, cultural considerations relate to issues of family support, trust, spirituality and religion, and unique distress reactions.

What follows are some cultural examples of these considerations; however, and as noted previously, we realize they cannot, nor are they intended to, capture the vast diversity of experience within cultural subgroups. So, again it is important for PFA providers to be open when working with different groups of people, ask questions when uncertain, and consult with others, and the literature, as needed.

Family Support and Trust

One of the more universal ethnocultural findings is that in the aftermath of critical incidents, family support, including from extended and collective family, plays an important role in fostering resilience (Carswell & Carswell, 2008; Ibrahim & Dykeman, 2011). In addition to maintaining close family ties, cultivating friendships and other close personal relationships that are predicated on respect, trust, genuine caring, and courage may be highly culturally valued (Arredondo, Bordes, & Paniagua, 2008). These qualities might be reflected and enhanced when providing PFA by initially asking about, and then showing respect for, the person's values, using "small talk" to help establish rapport. Recognize that extended greetings with physical closeness might occur (as may be the case in some Middle Eastern and Mediterranean cultures) and anticipate that sometimes those most impacted by critical incidents may demonstrate more concern and caring for others, including their children and parents, than for themselves, although this is not necessarily culturally bound (Abi-Hashem, 2008; Arredondo, Bordes, & Paniagua, 2008).

As noted, a PFA provider should also be sensitive to, and if uncertain inquire about, unfamiliar customs. For example, ask about taking off your shoes when entering someone's home, regardless of culture. Be aware that in some cultures it is customary to keep both feet on the floor, not cross your legs, and not expose the bottom of your feet (Gammel, 2008). Some other cultural data a RAPID PFA provider might consider when assessing and providing intervention tactics (see chapters 6 and 8) comes from an empirical prospective heart study that reported stress was associated with increased smoking, more fat consumption, and reduced hours of sleep; yet stress was also surprisingly associated with reports of increased physical activity (Sims et al., 2017). So, even though there can be considerable individual variability in these behavioral customs, a PFA provider might benefit from being mindful of them.

It also is prudent as a PFA provider to be aware that compared to the Western notion of "self" that is more individualistic (one's needs are often put before the needs of the group to which they belong) and values concepts like autonomy, assertiveness, and independence, some Asian cultures have traditionally adhered to a notion of "self" that is collectivistic, meaning that it is family-based (one's behavior reflects upon the entire family) and is predicated on cooperation and adaptation within a social hierarchy that is meant to enhance harmony and strong feelings of responsibility and obligation (Ino & Glicken, 1999). This may affect one's willingness to accept outside assistance. Furthermore, when working with someone in the aftermath of a critical incident from a collectivistic perspective, the PFA provider might encounter individuals who present as stoic, pragmatic, and possibly self-restrained (Leong & Lee, 2008). From a tactical perspective, the PFA provider could benefit from mirroring a more task-oriented approach, so open-ended questions and questions related to affect may not be as initially productive as questions that are more structured and problem-focused (Leong & Lee, 2008).

As already alluded to, one of the unique and ongoing tasks of PFA providers is to foster awareness about how their own cultural background can possibly impact their work with others. One of the most florid instances of this concept is the challenge sometimes associated with developing trust. People usually trust their families yet often have reasonable and understandable skepticism when considering allowing others into their community. Based on Maslow's (1970) seminal theory of hierarchy of needs, safety is considered the most basic psychological need (see chapter 7). So, as a PFA provider the effectiveness of your intervention often rests on working to establish safety, which in turn fosters trust.

There are many issues that can affect establishing trust in all cultures, such as living in rural areas, as noted previously. However, some of the more empirical and salient considerations related to the challenges in developing trust have been observed in the African American culture. Consider, for example, a study that has shown that African Americans, compared to Asians and Hispanics, report significantly higher perceptions of racial discrimination (Chou, Asnaani, & Hofmann, 2012), which, of course, could lead to feelings of mistrust regarding outsiders. In addition, trust of outsiders could be impacted by the highly publicized and notably wide racial divide that occurred following Hurricane Katrina in 2005, in which African Americans were documented to be disproportionate victims of the storm (Sherman & Shapiro, 2005). Moreover, African Americans reported significantly more anger and depression following the hurricane than did Whites and were four times more likely than Whites to report that the government's response would have been faster had the victims been White (White et al., 2007). Potentially exacerbating a sense of mistrust, and also related to traumatic events, are other data that note that mortality rates due to the use of lethal force by US police is 2.8 times higher for African American than White individuals (Buehler, 2017). In addition, the death of George Floyd on May 25, 2020, sparked national and international protests against police brutality, especially toward Black people.

Depending on the type of critical incident and its location, a RAPID PFA provider, particularly if considered an outsider to the community, should be aware of the possibility of initial mistrust when responding. The RAPID PFA provider should respect individuals' privacy and, as noted, expect some initial amount of scrutiny when working to establish rapport. However, trust can be facilitated by being open, honest, and clear in the explanation of the purpose of PFA; by answering questions; and, as noted, by inquiring about customs in which they are unaware.

Spirituality and Religion

Another seemingly cultural universal in the aftermath of critical incidents is the influence of spirituality and religion. While these terms are interrelated, spirituality generally refers to one's personal connection to larger perceived realities, including the material universe, whereas religion is considered to formalize these experiences (Josephson & Peteet, 2004).

Religious faith may play a central role in how survivors understand and cope with the adversity of trauma and disaster. The PFA provider is well-advised to determine what, if any, role spirituality and religion play in the felt experience of adversity. Some cultures have been noted, for example, to embrace religion and spirituality more so than other cultures (Taylor & Chatters, 2010), and the house of worship often serves as the epicenter of many communities. It is not surprising that during times of distress many religiously centric communities have been known to seek support through family members, community elders, or through spiritual or religious guidance or prayer and that these beliefs have been shown in some instances to decrease the community's willingness to seek outside mental health care (Rosales & Calvo, 2017). An example of instead seeking internal support comes from traditional spiritual leaders in the Islam religion, known as *imams*, who were shown to be essential in promoting mental health in the Muslim community in New York following the September 11 attacks (Abu-Ras & Abu-Bader, 2008).

Given the prominent cultural role of spirituality and religion in the aftermath of traumatic events, it seems prudent, therefore, that PFA providers should consider coordinating their efforts, when appropriate, with community leaders and local houses of worship (Paniagua, 2005). A successful model of this approach was when the Johns Hopkins Bloomberg School of Public Health recognized members of the faith-based community as being such an effective and valuable resource following critical incidents that the faith-based responders were provided PFA training to enhance their awareness of common physical and psychological responses to critical incidents as well as their role as spiritual communities in public health emergencies (Mc-Cabe et al., 2008; McCabe et al., 2014).

Distress Reactions

PFA providers will also benefit from understanding more about some of the cultural contexts of illness experiences and reactions (such as grief, mourning, and other specific illness symptoms), although there will be considerable variability among individual cultures. For example, although the distinction between grief and mourning may not apply to all cultures, the term *grief* has typically been used to describe the myriad internal emotional or affective reactions to loss, usually of a loved one (DeSpelder & Strickland, 2015; Jeffreys, 2011; Shear, 2015), whereas *mourning* is widely considered the public display of grief that is thought to be "shaped by the (often religious) beliefs and practices of a given society or cultural group" (Stroebe et al., 2008, p. 5). Regardless of the terms used, yet particularly relevant for this chapter, references and knowledge about grief are all considered culturally based (Rosenblatt, 2008). Therefore, some distinctive grief and mourning reactions from cultures that PFA providers might encounter following loss are worth noting.

For instance, visions of or hearing from the deceased as part of the grieving process is considered normative in many cultures and is typically not thought of as indicative of a pathological reaction (Simon, 2012). Another consideration is that in some Chinese cultures, 100 days of mourning after the death of a loved one, including not participating in parties, weddings, or other celebrations, occurs (Braun & Nichols, 1997). In the Mexican and Mexican American communities, the observation of Día de los Muertos (the Day of the Dead) is a three-day celebration beginning on October 31 that welcomes the deceased back into families because spirits of departed are believed to reenter the world (Norget, 2005). Moreover, in an empirical study comparing African American and Caucasian participants' grief reactions, results revealed that African Americans reported stronger bonds (i.e., some sort of contact) with the deceased, more distress over loss of an extended family member, less willingness to talk about the loss, and less likelihood to seek professional emotional health services (Laurie & Neimeyer, 2008).

In some extreme cases, and as noted in the cultural concepts of distress section of *DSM-5* (American Psychiatric Association, 2013), the syndrome *ataque de nervios* ("attack of nerves") may occur among Latinx. This syndrome, which most often results following a traumatic event relating to a family member, including death, entails a general sense of being out of control and may include screaming and shouting uncontrollably along with depersonalization and seizure-like behaviors. This symptom complex, which has been noted to occur more in females, is considered a more inclusive version of a panic attack (Lewis-Fernández et al., 2002; Liebowitz et al., 1994). As noted in chapter 3, managing an acute panic attack can be a challenge for a PFA provider; therefore, for those displaying the extreme symptoms described here, it may be prudent to attempt to get them to the next level of care.

Similar to *ataque de nervios, shenjing shuairuo*, which roughly translates to "weakness of the nervous system" in Mandarin Chinese, is a cultural syndrome that integrates traditional Chinese medicine with the Western diagnostic concept of neurasthenia that was used most widely in the latter part of the nineteenth century and introduced into China in the 1920s. Neurasthenia was a condition that included symptoms of fatigue, loss of motivation and concentration, and vague feelings of general unhappiness, or what we now euphemistically refer to as stress (Segen, 2006). Moreover, variants of the term neurasthenia, such as "combat neurasthenia" and "traumatic neurosis," serve as precursors to what we now know as posttraumatic stress disorder (PTSD) (Compston, 2013; Jones & Wessely, 2006).

Other neurasthenia-spectrum phenomena, such as *shinkei-suijaku* in Japan and *ashaktapanna* in India, exist, but *shenjing shuairuo* is noted prominently in the cultural concept of distress in *DSM-5* (American Psychiatric Association, 2013). *Shenjing shuairuo*, which does not have an organic cause, also remains within the *Chinese Classification of Mental Disorders* (Chinese Society of Psychiatry, 2001) and is associated with persistent mental and physical fatigue after exertion; irritability; excitability; physical discomfort (e.g., headaches, chest tightness); sleep disturbances; and secondary symptoms that include dizziness, memory problems, gastrointestinal problems, and sexual dysfunction. Precipitating events for symptoms of *shenjing shuairuo* include extreme psychosocial stressors, such as work or family-related distress, an acute sense of failure, or grief (Lewis-Fernández, Guarnaccia, & Ruiz, 2009). For a RAPID PFA provider it is worth noting that "the link between traumatic experiences and *shenjing shuairuo* reaching a threshold of clinical concern and impairment has long been recognized" (Hall et al., 2018, p. 737), and referrals to the next level of care should be considered if the reactions are extreme and persistent.

Another finding worth noting, and one associated with stigma, is that reporting mental health issues in some cultures may be considered shameful, so emotional symptoms might be described as physical symptoms (Al-Krenawi, 2005; Draguns, 1996; El-Islam, 2008; Leong & Lee, 2008; Zaroff et al., 2012). In addition to avoiding stigma associated with reporting psychological distress, physical symptom expression might be associated with a general help-seeking style (e.g., maintaining social connections that are consistent with a collectivistic culture), or it may simply be that some cultures give more credibility to somatic symptoms than psychological symptoms (Karasz, Dempsey, & Fallek, 2007; Zaroff et al., 2012). Regardless of basis, a RAPID PFA provider should ask about or listen for somatic symptoms as indications of signs of distress.

KEY POINT SUMMARY

The purpose of this chapter is to raise cultural awareness and cultural competency in PFA providers working with diverse people. We acknowledge and have emphasized that individuals receiving help are the ultimate authority on the formation and meaning of their culture. Given these caveats, let us review the main points of the chapter.

1. Culture is the lens through which members of a group experience shared knowledge, beliefs, morals, and customs.

2. PFA providers should work to enhance their cultural competency, which is meant to facilitate interacting with other people and is based on fostering openness, trust, and social justice. This enhancement is based on PFA providers exploring their own worldviews, beliefs, and possible biases and appreciating that differences among members of a cultural group may be as varied as differences between groups.

3. When initiating care, RAPID PFA providers should consider a person or community's preferred language (including sign language) and the location of the critical incident.

4. The importance of family, including extended family, is paramount in most cultures. It is helpful for PFA providers to understand the nuances associated with family, such as differences between individualistic and collectivistic cultures.

5. If a PFA provider is considered a cultural outsider, an initial amount of mistrust and skepticism can be expected, but openness, honesty, clearly describing the purpose of PFA, and inquiring about customs in which they are unaware are helpful to establish rapport.

6. Spirituality and religion are prominent resources in the aftermath of critical incidents, and PFA providers should consider coordinating their efforts, when appropriate, with community leaders and local houses of worship.

7. It is worthwhile for PFA providers to be aware of specific grief reactions that are considered normative in some cultures, such as visions of or hearing from the deceased. More extreme cultural reactions to critical incidents, such as *ataque de nervios* ("attack of nerves") in the Hispanic culture and *shenjing shuairuo* ("weakness of the nervous system" and predicated on the Western construct of neurasthenia) may occur.

References

Abi-Hashem, N. (2008). Arab Americans: Understanding their challenges, needs, and struggles. In A. J. Marsella, J. L. Johnson, P. Watson, &
J. Gryczynski (Eds.), *Ethnocultural perspectives on disaster and trauma* (pp.
115–173). New York, NY: Springer Science+Business Media.

Abu-Ras, W., & Abu-Bader, S. H. (2008). The impact of the September 11,
2001, attacks on the well-being of Arab Americans in New York City. *Journal of Muslim Mental Health, 3,* 217–239. http://dx.doi.org/10
.1080/15564900802487634.

Al-Krenawi, A. (2005). Mental health practice in Arab countries. *Current
Opinion in Psychiatry, 18,* 560–564. http://dx.doi.org/10.1097/01.yco.0000
179498.46182.8b.

American Psychiatric Association (2013). *Diagnostic and statistical manual
of mental disorders* (5th ed.). Washington, DC: American Psychiatric Association.

Arredondo, P., Bordes, V., & Paniagua, F. A. (2008). Mexican, Mexican
Americans, Caribbean, and Other Latin Americans. In A. J. Marsella,
J. L. Johnson, P. Watson, & J. Gryczynski (Eds.), *Ethnocultural perspectives
on disaster and trauma* (pp. 299–320). New York, NY: Springer Science+
Business Media.

Barzinpour, F., & Esmaeili, V. (2014). A multi-objective relief chain location
distribution model for urban disaster management. *International Journal of
Advanced Manufacturing Technology, 70,* 1291–1302. http://dx.doi.org/10
.1007/s00170-013-5379-x.

Braun, K. L., & Nichols, R. (1997). Death and dying in four Asian-American
cultures: A descriptive study. *Death Studies, 21,* 327–359. http://dx.doi.org
/10.1080/074811897201877.

Buehler, J. W. (2017). Racial/ethnic disparities in the use of lethal force by
US police, 2010–2014. *American Journal of Public Health, 107,* 295–297.
http://dx.doi.org/10.2105/AJPH.2016.303575.

Carswell, S. B., & Carswell, M. A. (2008). Meeting the physical, psychological, and social needs of African Americans following a disaster. In A. J.
Marsella, J. L. Johnson, P. Watson, & J. Gryczynski (Eds.), *Ethnocultural
perspectives on disaster and trauma* (pp. 39–71). New York, NY: Springer
Science+Business Media.

Chinese Society of Psychiatry. (2001). *The Chinese classification of mental
disorders* (3rd ed. [CCMD-3]). [In Chinese]. Shandong, China: Shandong
Publishing House of Science and Technology.

Chou, T., Asnaani, A., & Hofmann, S. G. (2012). Perception of racial discrimination and psychopathology across three US ethnic minority groups. *Culture Diversity & Ethnic Minority Psychology, 18,* 74–81. http://dx.doi.org/10.1037/a0025432.

Compston, A. (2013). From the archives: War-neurasthenia, acute and chronic. *Brain, 136,* 1681–1686. http://dx.doi.org/10.1093/brain/awt136.

Despeaux, K. E., Lating, J. M., Everly, G. S., Jr., Sherman, M. F., & Kirkhart, M. W. (2019). A randomized controlled trial assessing the efficacy of group psychological first aid. *Journal of Nervous and Mental Disease, 207,* 626–632. http://dx.doi.org/10.1097/NMD.0000000000001029.

DeSpelder, L. A., & Strickland, A. L. (2015). *The last dance: Encountering death and dying* (10th ed.). New York, NY: McGraw Hill.

Draguns, J. G. (1996). Abnormal behaviour in Chinese societies: Clinical, epidemiological, and comparative studies, In M. H. Bond (Ed.), *Handbook of Chinese psychology* (pp. 412–418). Hong Kong: Oxford University Press.

El-Islam, M. F. (2008). Arab culture and mental health care. *Transcultural Psychiatry, 45,* 671–682. http://dx.doi.org/10.1177/1363461508100788.

Forbes, D., Lewis, V., Varker, T., Phelps, A., O'Donnell, M., Wade, D. J., . . . Creamer, M. (2011). Psychological first aid following trauma: Implementation and evaluation framework for high-risk organizations. *Psychiatry, 74,* 224–239. http://dx.doi.org/10.1521/psyc.2011.74.3.224.

Freire, P. (1973). *Education for critical consciousness.* New York, NY: Seabury Press.

Gammel, C. (2008, December 15). Arab culture: The insult of the shoe. *The Telegraph.* https://www.telegraph.co.uk/news/worldnews/middleeast/iraq/3776970/Arab-culture-the-insult-of-the-shoe.html.

Hall, B. J., Change, K., Chen, W., Sou, K. L., Latkin, C., & Yeung, A. (2018). Exploring the association between depression and *shenjing shuairuo* in a population representative epidemiological study of Chinese adults in Guangzhou, China. *Transcultural Psychiatry, 55,* 733–753. http://dx.doi.org/10.1177/1363461518778670.

Halpern, J., & Tramontin, M. (2007). *Disaster mental health: Theory and practice.* Belmont, CA: Thompson Brooks / Cole Publishing.

Ibrahim, F. A., & Dykeman, C. (2011). Counseling Muslim Americans: Cultural and spiritual assessments. *Journal of Counseling & Development, 89,* 387–396. http://dx.doi.org/10.1002/j.1556-6676.2011.tb02835.x.

Ino, S. M., & Glicken, M. D. (2010). Treating Asian American clients in crisis: A collectivist approach. *Smith College Studies in Social Work, 69,* 525–540. http://dx.doi.org/10.1080/00377319909517572.

Jeffreys, J. S. (2011). *Helping grieving people: When tears are not enough* (2nd ed.). New York, NY: Routledge.

Jones, W., & Wessely, S. (2006). Psychological trauma: A historical perspective. *Psychiatry, 5,* 217–220. http://dx.doi.org/10.1053/j.mppsy.2006.04.011.

Josephson, A. M., & Peteet, J. R. (Eds.). (2004). *Handbook of spirituality and worldview in clinical practice.* Arlington, VA: American Psychiatric Publishing.

Kagawa-Singer, M., Dressler, W. W., George, S. M., & Elwood, W. N. (2014). *The cultural framework for health: An integrative approach for research and program design and evaluation.* Bethesda, MD: National Institutes of Health.

Karasz, A., Dempsey, K., & Fallek, R. (2007). Cultural differences in the experience of everyday symptoms: A comparative study of South Asia and European American women. *Culture, Medicine and Psychiatry, 31,* 473–497. http://dx.doi.org/10.1007/s11013-007-9066-y.

Laurie, A., & Neimeyer, R. A. (2008). African Americans in bereavement: Grief as a function of ethnicity. *OMEGA, 57,* 173–193. http://dx.doi.org/10.2190/OM.57.2.d.

Leong, F. T. L., & Lee, S-H. (2008). Chinese Americans: Guidelines for disaster mental health workers. In A. J. Marsella, J. L. Johnson, P. Watson, & J. Gryczynski (Eds.), *Ethnocultural perspectives on disaster and trauma* (pp. 241–269). New York, NY: Springer Science+Business Media.

Lewis-Fernández, R., Guarnaccia, P. J., Martínez, I. E., Salmán, E., Schmidt, A., & Liebowitz, M. (2002). Comparative phenomenology of *ataques de nervios,* panic attacks, and panic disorder. *Culture, Medicine, and Psychiatry, 26,* 199–223. http://dx.doi.org/10.1023/A:1016349624867.

Lewis-Fernández, R., Guarnaccia, P. J., & Ruiz, P. (2009). Culture-bound syndromes. In B. J. Sadock, V. A. Sadock, & P. Ruiz (Eds.), *Kaplan & Sadock's comprehensive textbook of psychiatry* (9th ed., Vol. II, pp. 2519–2538). New York, NY: Lippincott Williams & Wilkins.

Liebowitz, M. R., Salmán, E., Jusino, C. M., Garfunkel, R., Street, L., Cárdenas, D. L., . . . Davies, S. (1994). *Ataque de nervios* and panic disorder. *American Journal of Psychiatry, 151,* 871–875. http://dx.doi.org/10.1176/ajp.151.6.871.

Lopez, Leo, III, Hart, L. H., III, & Katz, M. H. (2021). Racial and ethnic health disparities related to COVID-19. *JAMA, 325,* 719–720. http://dx.doi.org/10.1001/jama.2020.26443.

Maslow, A. H. (1970). *Motivation and personality.* New York, NY: Harper & Row.

McCabe, O. L., Mosley, A. M., Gwon, H. S., Everly, G. S., Lating, J. M., Links, J. M., & Kaminsky, M. J. (2008). The tower of ivory meets the house of worship: Psychological first aid training for the faith community. *International Journal of Emergency Mental Health, 9*, 171–180.

McCabe, O. L., Semon, N. L., Lating, J. M., Everly, G. S., Jr., Perry, C. J., Moore, S. S., . . . Links, J. M. (2014). An academic-government-faith partnership to build disaster mental health preparedness and community resilience. *Public Health Reports, 129*(Suppl 4), 96–106. http://dx.doi.org/10.1177/003335 49141296S413.

Norget, K. (2005). *Days of death, days of life: Ritual in the popular culture of Oaxaca.* New York, NY: Columbia University Press.

Ogburn, W. F. (1966). *Social change with respect to cultural and original nature.* New York, NY: Dell Publishing.

Paniagua, F. A. (2005). *Assessing and treating culturally diverse clients: A practical guide.* Thousand Oaks, CA: Sage.

Pederson, P. (1987). Ten frequent assumptions of cultural bias in counseling. *Journal of Multicultural Counseling and Development, 15*, 16–24. http://dx.doi .org/10.1002/j.2161-1912.1987.tb00374.x.

Riding-Malon, R., & Werth, J. L. (2014). Psychological practice in rural settings: At the cutting edge. *Professional Psychology: Research and Practice, 45*, 85–91. http://dx.doi.org/10.1037/a0036172.

Rosales, R., & Calvo, R. (2017). *"Si Dios Quiere"*: Fatalismo and the use of mental health services among Latinos with a history of depression. *Social Work in Health Care, 56*, 748–764. http://dx.doi.org/10.1080/00981389.2017 .1339760.

Rosenblatt, P. C. (2008). Grief across cultures: A review and research agenda. In M. S. Stroebe, R. O. Hansson, H. Schut, & W. Stroebe (Eds.), *Handbook of bereavement research and practice: Advances in theory and intervention* (pp. 207–222). Washington, DC: American Psychological Association Press. http://dx.doi.org/10.1037/14498-010.

Roysircar, G. (2004). Child survivor of war: A case study. *Journal of Multicultural Counseling and Development, 32*, 168–180. http://dx.doi.org/10.1002 /j.2161-1912.2004.tb00369.x.

Segen, J. C. (2006). *Concise dictionary of modern medicine.* New York, NY: McGraw-Hill.

Shear, M. K. (2015). Complicated grief. *New England Journal of Medicine, 372*, 153–160. http://dx.doi.org/10.1056/NEJMcp1315618.

Sherman, A., & Shapiro, I. (2005). *Essential facts about the victims of Hurricane Katrina*. Washington, DC: Center on Budget and Policy Priorities.

Simon, D. L. (2012). Religious visions and voices. In C. Murray (Ed.), *Mental health and anomalous experience*, (pp. 19–32). Hauppauge, NY: Nova Science Publishers.

Sims, M., Lipford, K.J., Patel, N., Ford, C. D., Min, Y. I., & Wyatt, S. B. (2017). Psychosocial factors and behaviors in African Americans: The Jackson Heart Study. *American Journal of Preventive Medicine, 52*, S48–S55. http://dx .doi.org/10.1016/j.amepre.2016.09.020.

Stroebe, M. S., Hansson, R. O., Schut, H., & Stroebe, W. (2008). Bereavement research: Contemporary perspectives. In M. S. Stroebe, H. Hansson, W. Schut, & W. Stroebe (Eds.), *Handbook of bereavement research and practice: Advances in theory and intervention* (pp. 3–25). Washington, DC: American Psychological Association Press. http://dx.doi.org/10.1037/14498-001.

Sue, D. W., Arredondo, P., & McDavis, R. J. (1992). Multicultural counseling competencies and standards: A call to the profession. *Journal of Multicultural Counseling and Development, 20*, 64–88. http://dx.doi.org/10.1002 /j.2161-1912.1992.tb00563.x.

Taylor, R., & Chatters, L. M. (2010). Importance of religion and spirituality in the lives of African Americans, Caribbean Blacks and non-Hispanic Whites. *Journal of Negro Education, 79*, 280–294.

TeachMideast. (n.d). Arab, Middle Eastern, and Muslim? What's the difference?! Retrieved May 11, 2020, from https://teachmideast.org/articles/arab -middle-eastern-and-muslim-whats-the-difference.

Triandis, H. C. (2007). *Culture and psychology: A history of the study of their relationship*. New York: NY: Guilford Press.

Turley, A. C. (2016). *Urban culture: Exploring cities and cultures*. London, England: Routledge.

Tylor, E. B. (1871). *Primitive culture: Researches into the development of mythology, philosophy, religion, art, and custom* (Vol. 1). London, England: John Murray.

Watts, R. J., Diemer, M. A., & Voight, A. M. (2011). Critical consciousness: Current status and future directions. *New Directions for Child and Adolescent Development*, no. 134, 43–57. http://dx.doi.org/10.1002/cd.310.

Weaver, H. N., & Wodarski, J. S. (1995). Cultural issues in crisis intervention: Guidelines for culturally competent practice. *Family Therapy, 22*, 213–223.

West-Olatunji, C., & Yoon, E. (2013). Culture-centered perspectives on disaster and crisis counseling. *Journal of Asia Pacific Counseling, 3*, 35–43. http://dx.doi.org/10.18401/2013.3.1.3.

Whaley, A. L., & Davis, K. E. (2007). Cultural competence and evidence-based practice in mental health services: A complementary perspective. *American Psychologist, 62*, 563–574. http://dx.doi.org/10.1037/0003-066X .62.6.563.

White, I. K., Philpot, T. S, Wylie, K., & McGowen, E. (2007). Feeling the pain of my people: Hurricane Katrina, racial inequality, and the psyche of Black America. *Journal of Black Studies, 37*, 523–538. http://dx.doi.org/10.1177 /0021934706296191.

Zaroff, C. M., Davis, M. J., Chio, P. H., & Madhavan, D. (2012). Somatic presentations of distress in China. *Australian and New Zealand Journal of Psychiatry, 46*, 1053–1057. http://dx.doi.org/10.1177/0004867412450077.

TWELVE | Expanding Surge Capacity

Strengthening the Fabric of Community
Mental Health Services

IN THE EARLY 1990S, I (GSE) was invited to give a presentation to Red Cross disaster response volunteers in a small city in Iowa. I was asked to provide training in basic psychological crisis intervention with an emphasis on assisting individuals in crisis using the fundamentals of psychological first aid (PFA). Prior to the training I was invited to the monthly meeting of the community mental health consortium. There were representatives from traditional mental health agencies and from social work, psychological, and psychiatric professions as expected. I was surprised, however, to also see representatives from various disaster response agencies, as well as the law enforcement, fire service, and emergency medicine professions. This amalgam of disaster and emergency responders were at these meetings, not because of their training in emergency and disaster response per se, but rather they were there because these emergency responders made up much of the volunteer crisis outreach and mobile crisis intervention capacity in this community. They were a formal and integral part of this community's overall mental health initiative. They were ideally suited to provide psychological crisis services because not only were they trained in emergency response by virtue of their professional roles but they also knew the community very well and, most importantly, they had all received specialized psychological crisis intervention training. These emergency services professionals represented a core element in the overall fabric of their community's mental health services. In doing so, they greatly expanded the overall mental health capacity of their community and could play an especially useful role in enhancing surge capacity should a disaster occur. In this chapter we examine PFA at this crucial community level.

The Need To Expand Mental Health Capacity Using Nontraditional Models

Daniel Levine (2018), writing for *US News and World Reports*, underscores disturbing trends that have been known yet remain largely unaddressed. He reports,

> Two disturbing trend lines are currently crossing in the area of mental health care. One line, tracking demand for such care, is rapidly rising. In the US, nearly 1 in 5 people has some sort of mental health condition according to the *Journal of the American Medical Association*. The disease burden—the impact of a health problem as measured by financial cost, death rates, disability, and other measures—of mental health and substance use disorders was higher than for any other condition in 2015, *JAMA* reported.
>
> The other trend line, measuring the number of mental health care providers in practice, is barely holding steady. A 2016 report released by the Health Resources and Services Administration projected the supply of workers in selected behavioral health professions to be approximately 250,000 workers short of the projected demand in 2025.

To Levine's second point, as of March 2021, there were over 3,400 areas in the United States designated as "underserved" (Health Resources and Services Administration, 2021).

In early 2020, the United Nations warned of an impending mental health crisis resulting from COVID-19: "Many people who previously coped well, are now less able to cope because of the multiple stressors generated by the pandemic. And those who previously had a mental health condition, may experience a worsening of their condition and reduced functioning" (p. 6). The United Nations report emphasized the mental health challenges to frontline responders and health care professionals, noting they are at high risk for psychological injury. And the *New York Times* referred to the mental health challenges as a "parallel pandemic" (Jacobs, 2021). In support of this notion, and as noted in chapter 3, a national survey conducted during the COVID-19 pandemic that included 1,441 respondents revealed the prevalence of depression symptoms was more than threefold higher during the pandemic than before it (Ettman et al., 2020).

In the influential report *The State of Mental Health in America* (Reinert, Nguyen, & Fritze, 2021), published by the nonprofit foundation Mental Health America (formerly known as the National Mental Health Association), the following trends were revealed:

- Prior to COVID-19, the prevalence of mental illness among adults was increasing, with 19% of adults in the United States experiencing a mental disorder in 2017–2018.
- The number of people screening with moderate to severe symptoms of depression and anxiety increased during the pandemic surge and was at least 30% higher than rates prior to COVID-19.
- Since March 2020, more than 178,000 people have reported frequent suicidal ideation.
- Almost 10% of youth surveyed expressed signs of depression, which is a worsening trend.
- Loneliness or isolation are conditions fueling depression.

The US Census Bureau (2021) also described COVID-related data wherein 41% of adults reported symptoms of anxiety or depression during the second winter (i.e., January–March 2021) of the pandemic.

Generally speaking, in the wake of any adversity (e.g., disaster, disease, violence), it is a truism that there will be more psychological "casualties" than physical casualties (Bass, Azur, & Person, 2005; Institute of Medicine, 2003; Lating, 2005). Simply said, the mental health surge (increased need for psychological support services) will often be greater than the physical health surge. Pioneer disaster psychiatrist Beverley Raphael (1986) estimated that about 25% of a population affected by disaster would suffer from psychological distress and dysfunction, what she referred to as "disaster syndrome." Norris et al. (2002), in a review of 160 studies covering 60,000 survivors, concluded that roughly 25% to 60% of those impacted by disaster (including mass violence) would suffer severe to very severe impairment with the adverse impact being most significant in developing nations.

In response to mass violence and terrorism perpetrated within the United States, Everly et al. (2005) estimated almost two decades ago that the point prevalence of posttraumatic stress (substantial stress symptomatology) ranged from 16% to 45% for adults. The time interval for these assessments ranged from several days post event to about six months. The point prevalence of probable posttraumatic stress disorder (PTSD) was estimated to range from 7.5% to 34% for those samples derived from targeted cities or populations. For those most directly exposed, the point prevalence of PTSD ranged from 28% to 34% within samples where assessments were conducted within six months of the event, to 13% to 18% within samples where assessments were conducted a year or more after the event.

Areas compounding the public health burden of providing services to the mental health surge are (1) those where access to formal mental services has been compromised and (2) otherwise underserved places (rural areas, developing nations, geographically isolated areas). This reality has been daunting for public health planners even under the best of circumstances in otherwise resource-rich environments, such as in most of North America. Disasters accentuate these problems. Even in the best of times, many individuals resist seeking psychological support. In some instances, there may be mistrust of the mental health community. In others, there may be stigma. Of course, these barriers are compounded to a greater degree in the latter, underserved low-resource areas.

Using PFA to Expand Community Psychological
Support Capacity

In their monograph *Health Care at the Crossroads*, the Joint Commission on Accreditation of Healthcare Organizations (2003) defined *surge capacity* as "the ability to expand care capabilities in response to sudden or more prolonged demand" (p. 19). They further indicate that surge capacity "is perhaps the most fundamental component of an emergency preparedness program" (p. 19). In anticipation of a continuing trend of disasters and community emergencies, the need to increase psychological surge capacity becomes self-evident. Certainly, there is no debate on the need to enhance mental health capacity for the over 3,400 areas in the United States that are considered underserved. However, the need to expand continual access to psychological support throughout all communities, perhaps even approximating universal psychological health care, should now be self-evident. The challenge is how to best do so. Reliance upon traditional mental health services is simply not an option in the wake of community adversity or large-scale human suffering. Access to trained mental health providers is limited during those chaotic times, and even more so in geographically isolated areas or developing nations. To remedy this problem, recommendations from the Johns Hopkins Center for Public Health Preparedness have included the training of local human resources to provide psychological support and "microcounseling" to enhance community resilience (Everly & Parker, 2005; Everly, 2020a, 2020b; McCabe et al., 2014). Microcounseling was originally a method for teaching introductory counseling skills (Ivey et al., 1968), but we use the term here to refer to the aggregation of those basic skills as applied in brief episodic crisis-oriented interactions.

As noted in earlier chapters, historically, community-based crisis intervention initiatives have been shown to be effective in fostering resilience by reducing the number of frank psychiatric cases, facilitating access to more traditional psychological care when needed, and sustaining compliance to treatment (Bordow & Porritt, 1979; Bunn & Clarke, 1979; Decker & Stubblebine, 1972; Langsley, Machotka, & Flomenhaft, 1971; Parad, 1971; Parad & Parad, 1968a, 1968b). Also in earlier chapters, we touted the demonstrated ability of community peer/paraprofessionals to provide effective psychological support in times of crisis and otherwise. Might this be a model that could be employed to increase the availability of psychological services?

Civilian paraprofessionals, educators, faith-based leaders, and emergency services personnel have been successfully trained to deliver brief counseling and psychological crisis intervention services since the 1960s, and the provision of such training has been the expressed mission of the United Nations–affiliated nonprofit organization International Critical Incident Stress Foundation since the late 1980s (Brown, 1974; Defense Centers of Excellence, 2011; Department of Justice, 2019; Eisdorpher & Golann, 1969; Everly & Kennedy, 2019; Everly et al., 2014; Greenstone, 2005; Hattie, Sharpley, & Rogers, 1984; Ivey et al., 1968; Jain, 2010; Levenson, 2003; Noullet et al., 2018). In an early compelling review, Durlak (1979) analyzed all published studies that had compared the clinical outcomes of mental health professionals (such as psychologists, psychiatrists, and social workers) with those of peer/paraprofessionals. The results of his analysis of 42 research studies revealed the effectiveness of volunteer peer/paraprofessionals was overall comparable to trained mental health professionals and, in some studies, superior to the professionals. Durlak concluded, "Professional mental health education training and experience are not necessary prerequisites for an effective helping person" (p. 6).

Dr. Gerald Jacobs (2016), a pioneer in disaster mental health, also advocates for the creation of the capacity to provide PFA at the community level. He notes his work on community-based PFA was initiated in Denmark and subsequently evolved into his current recommendations. He emphasizes one does not need to be a mental health clinician to provide effective psychological support. In his book *Community-Based Psychological First Aid* he suggests active listening, problem-solving, stress management, and knowing when to seek higher levels of care as fundamental skills in community PFA that can be acquired without attaining licensure in a mental health profession.

Cherie Castellano at Rutgers University received the 2018 Silver Medal from the American Psychiatric Association in recognition of her success in implementing peer-based crisis intervention programs (Castellano, 2012, 2018; Evans et al., 2020). The interventionists who staffed her programs were community-based civilians and uniformed emergency services personnel (police, firefighters, etc.) specifically trained in the provision of psychological crisis intervention using highly structured intervention protocols.

Consistent with Ivey et al. (1968) and their concept of microcounseling, Stapleton et al. (2006) and Everly (2002) concluded that effectiveness seemed associated with following well-structured training and/ or intervention protocols. Simply speaking with a person in distress while hoping for a verbal "Hail Mary" seldom proves to be an adequate intervention. Building on the success of models such as Castellano's and Ivey's, it might be useful to develop a psychological analogue to the paramedicine concept of advanced life support by employing a model of integrated peer support (IPS). An IPS approach would consist of integrating peer psychological first aid (Everly et al., 2016; Noullet et al., 2018) with techniques such as Castellano's reciprocal peer support and Ivey's peer microcounseling. Analyses have documented the effectiveness of PFA and of reciprocal peer support (Everly et al., 2016; Evans et al., 2020). And the microcounseling method is a well-developed approach to training preprofessional and lay counselors (Ivey, 1970; Ivey et al., 1968). In this way, extending the theme of peer/paraprofessional training may hold potential for increasing community psychological support capacity overall.

The wisdom of expanding surge capacity and overall ongoing community mental health capacity using persons outside of the mental health professions should not be a stretch. It is prudent to remember Rapoport's (1965) assertion, "A little help, rationally directed and purposely focused at a strategic time, is more effective than extensive help given at a period of less emotional accessibility" (p. 30). A similar assertion regarding the effectiveness of compassionate and practical psychological support was made after September 11 (Bisson et al., 2007).

As support grows for the continued utilization of PFA, consideration should be made for its use beyond the initial formulated applications in disaster and crisis. PFA may be considered a psychological intervention designed to foster human resilience. As such, it fits nicely into the overall fabric of community psychological services. In the final analysis, consonant with World Health Organization (2018) goals and recommendations, PFA may even be used as an intervention to foster the achievement of universal mental health coverage delivered not only in nonspecialized health settings but via nontraditional community-based mechanisms as well. Furthermore, as noted in chapter 2, we endorse the use of PFA delivered using a virtual platform (akin to telehealth). Virtual PFA is consistent with the community model presented in this chapter as it can dramatically expand both the volume of services provided as well as the geographic regions covered.

KEY POINT SUMMARY

1. It is generally accepted that there is a shortage of psychological support services in much of the United States and North America.

2. In the wake of adversity, it is a truism that there will be more psychological "casualties" than physical casualties wherein the mental health surge will often be greater than the physical health surge.

3. Given a paucity of traditional mental health resources or logistical challenges in accessing those services, new models will need to be employed to best meet these challenges.

4. In crisis, that which is most needed is practical assistance delivered in a compassionate manner (Bisson et al., 2007).

5. Community-based crisis intervention initiatives have been shown to be effective in reducing psychiatric caseness, facilitating access to more traditional psychological care when needed, and sustaining compliance when in treatment (Bordow & Porritt, 1979; Bunn & Clarke, 1979; Decker & Stubblebine, 1972; Langsley, Machotka, & Flomenhaft, 1971; Parad, 1971; Parad & Parad, 1968a, 1968b).

6. Peer interventionists (community members from professions other than mental health) as the providers of such community crisis intervention services have been shown to be effective in delivering acute psychological support (Castellano, 2018; Defense Centers of Excellence, 2011; Durlak, 1979; Eisdorpher & Golann, 1969).

7. Psychological first aid (PFA) has been universally endorsed as an important addition to the corpus of mental health–related support services.

8. The notion of "integrated peer support" (IPS) may be one way of expanding capacity. IPS may be thought of as a combination of psychological first aid (Everly & Lating, 2017), reciprocal peer support and wellness (Castellano, 2012, 2018), and microcounseling (Ivey, 1970; Ivey et al., 1968), creating the psychological equivalent of the paramedicine concept of advanced life support.

9. PFA may be considered a psychological crisis intervention designed to foster human resilience.

10. Jacobs (2016), in his book *Community-Based Psychological First Aid*, advocates and provides guidance for establishing psychological support programs in communities. He suggests active listening, problem-solving, stress management, and knowing when to seek higher levels of care as fundamental skills in community PFA.

References

Bisson, J. I., Brayne, M., Ochberg, F., & Everly, G. S., Jr. (2007). Early psychosocial intervention following traumatic events. *American Journal of Psychiatry, 164*, 1016–1019. http://dx.doi.org/10.1176/ajp.2007.164.7.1016.

Bass, J., Azur, M., & Person, C. (2005). Mental health consequences of disaster. In G. S. Everly, Jr., and C. L. Parker (Eds.), *Mental health aspects of disaster: Public health preparedness and response* (pp. 18–44). Baltimore, MD: Johns Hopkins Center for Public Health Preparedness.

Bordow, S., & Porritt, D. (1979). An experimental evaluation of crisis intervention. *Social Science and Medicine, 13*, 251–256. http://dx.doi.org/10.1016/0271-7123(79)90042-7.

Brown, W. F. (1974). Effectiveness of paraprofessionals: The evidence. *Personnel and Guidance Journal, 53*, 257–264. http://dx.doi.org/10.1002/j.2164-4918.1974.tb03779.x.

Bunn, T., & Clarke, A. (1979). Crisis intervention: An experimental study of the effects of a brief period of counselling on the anxiety of relatives of seriously injured or ill hospital patients. *British Journal of Medical Psychology, 52*, 191–195. http://dx.doi.org/10.1111/j.2044-8341.1979.tb02514.x.

Castellano, C. (2012). Reciprocal peer support (RPS): A decade of not so random acts of kindness. *International Journal of Emergency Mental Health, 14*, 137–142.

Castellano, C. (2018). Silver award: Reciprocal peer support for addressing mental health crises among police, veterans, mothers of special needs children, and others. 2018 APA Psychiatric Services Achievement Awards. *Psychiatric Services, 69*, e7-8. http://dx.doi.org/10.1176/appi.ps.691006.

Decker, J., & Stubblebine, J. (1972). Crisis intervention and prevention of psychiatric disability: A follow-up study. *American Journal of Psychiatry, 129*, 725–729. http://dx.doi.org/10.1176/ajp.129.6.725.

Defense Centers of Excellence (2011). *Best practices identified for peer support programs.* Washington, DC: Defense Centers of Excellence.

Department of Justice, Community Oriented Policing Services. (2019). *Law enforcement mental health and wellness act: Report to Congress.* Washington, DC: US Department of Justice.

Durlak, J. (1979). Comparative effectiveness of paraprofessional and professional helpers. *Psychological Bulletin, 86*, 80–92. http://dx.doi.org/10.1037/0033-2909.86.1.80.

Eisdorpher, C., & Golann, S. (1969). Principles for the training of "new professionals" in mental health. *Community Mental Health Journal, 5*, 349–357. http://dx.doi.org/10.1007/BF01438980.

Ettman, C. K., Abdalla S. M., Cohen, G. H., Sampson, L., Vivier, P. M., & Galea, S. (2020). Prevalence of depression symptoms in US adults before and during the COVID-19 pandemic. *JAMA Network Open, 3*, e2019686. http://dx.doi.org/10.1001/jamanetworkopen.2020.19686.

Evans, M., Tang, P.Y., Bhushan, N., Fisher, E. B., Dreyer, D., & Castellano, C. (2020). Standardization and adaptability for dissemination of telephone peer support for high-risk groups: General evaluation and lessons learned. *Translational Behavioral Medicine, 10*, 506–515. http://dx.doi.org/10.1093/tbm/ibaa047.

Everly, G. S., Jr. (2002). Thoughts on peer (paraprofessional) support in the provision of mental health services. *International Journal of Emergency Mental Health, 4*, 89–90.

Everly, G. S., Jr. (2020a). Psychological first aid (PFA) to expand mental health support and foster resiliency in underserved and access-compromised areas. *Crisis, Stress, and Human Resilience, 1*, 227–232.

Everly, G. S., Jr. (2020b). Psychological first aid to support healthcare professionals. *Journal of Patient Safety and Risk Management, 25*, 159–162. http://doi.org/10.1177/2516043520944637.

Everly, G. S., Jr., Barnett, D., Parker, C. L., & Links, J. (2005). *A review of the mental health consequences of terrorism in the United States.* Baltimore, MD: Johns Hopkins Center for Public Health Preparedness.

Everly, G. S., Jr., & Kennedy, C. (2019). Content validation of the Johns Hopkins model of psychological first aid (RAPID-PFA) expanded curriculum. *Crisis, Stress, and Human Resilience, 1*, 6–14.

Everly, G. S., Jr., & Lating, J. M. (2017). *The Johns Hopkins guide to psychological first aid.* 1st ed. Baltimore, MD: Johns Hopkins University Press.

Everly, G. S., Jr., Lating, J. M., Sherman, M., & Goncher, I. (2016). The potential efficacy of psychological first aid on self-reported anxiety and mood: A pilot study. *Journal of Nervous and Mental Disease, 204*, 233–235. http://dx.doi.org/10.1097/NMD.0000000000000429.

Everly, G. S., Jr., McCabe, O. L., Semon, N., Thompson, C. B., & Links, J. (2014). The development of a model of psychological first aid for non-mental health trained public health personnel: The Johns Hopkins RAPID-PFA. *Journal of Public Health Management and Practice, 20*, S24–S29. http://dx.doi.org/10.1097/PHH.0000000000000065.

Everly, G. S., Jr., & Parker, C. L. (Eds.) (2005). *Mental health aspects of disaster: Public health preparedness and response.* Baltimore, MD: Johns Hopkins Center for Public Health Preparedness.

Greenstone, J. L. (2005). Peer support for police hostage and crisis negotiators. *Journal of Police Crisis Negotiations, 5*, 45–55. http://dx.doi.org/10.1300/J173v05n01_05.

Hattie, J. A., Sharpley, C. F., & Rogers, H. J. (1984). Comparative effectiveness of professional and paraprofessional helpers. *Psychological Bulletin, 95*, 534–541. http://dx.doi.org/10.1037/0033-2909.95.3.534.

Health Resources and Services Administration (2016). *National projections of supply and demand for selected behavioral health practitioners: 2013-2025.* Rockville, Maryland: National Center for Health Workforce Analysis. https://bhw.hrsa.gov/sites/default/files/bureau-health-workforce/data-research/behavioral-health-2013-2025.pdf.

Health Resources and Services Administration (2021, February). *Shortage areas.* https://data.hrsa.gov/topics/health-workforce/shortage-areas.

Institute of Medicine. (2003). *Preparing for the psychological consequences of terrorism: A public health strategy.* Washington, DC: National Academy of Sciences.

Ivey, A. E. (1970). Attending behavior: The basis of counseling. *School Psychologist, 18,* 117–119. http://www.jstor.org/stable/23896657.

Ivey, A. E., Normington, C., Miller, C.D., Morrill, W., & Haase, R.F. (1968). Microcounseling and attending behavior. *Journal of Counseling Psychology, 15,* 1–12. http://dx.doi.org/10.1037/h0026129.

Jacobs, A. (2021, February 5). One year in, pandemic pushes health care workers to the brink. *New York Times,* Section A, p. 6.

Jacobs, G. A. (2016). *Community-based psychological first aid.* New York, NY: Butterworth-Heineman.

Jain, S. (2010). The role of paraprofessionals in providing treatment for posttraumatic stress disorder in low-resource communities. *JAMA, 304,* 571–572. http://dx.doi.org/10.1001/jama.2010.1096.

Joint Commission on Accreditation of Healthcare Organizations. (2003). *Health care at the crossroads: Strategies for creating and sustaining community-wide emergency preparedness systems.* Oakbrook Terrace, IL: Joint Commission on Accreditation of Healthcare Organizations.

Langsley, D., Machotka, P., & Flomenhaft, K. (1971). Avoiding mental health admission: A follow-up. *American Journal of Psychiatry, 127,* 1391–1394. http://dx.doi.org/10.1176/ajp.127.10.1391.

Lating, J. M. (2005). Psychological contagion effect. In G. S. Everly, Jr., and C. L. Parker (Eds.), *Mental health aspects of disaster: Public health preparedness and response* (pp. 51–68). Baltimore, MD: Johns Hopkins Center for Public Health Preparedness.

Levine, D. (2018, May 25). What's the answer to the shortage of mental health care providers? *US News and World Reports.* https://health.usnews.com/health-care/patient-advice/articles/2018-05-25/whats-the-answer-to-the-shortage-of-mental-health-care-providers.

Levenson, R. (2003). Peer support in law enforcement. *International Journal of Emergency Mental Health, 5,* 147–152.

McCabe, O. L., Semon, N., Thompson, C. B., Lating, J. M., Everly, G. S., Jr., Perry, C. J., . . . Links, J. M. (2014). Building a national model of public mental health preparedness and community resilience: Validation of a dual-intervention, systems-based approach. *Disaster Medicine and Public Health Preparedness, 8,* 511–526. http://dx.doi.org/10.1017/dmp.2014.119.

Norris, F. H., Friedman, M. J., Watson, P. J., Byrne, C. M., Diaz, E., & Kaniasty, K. (2002). 60,000 disaster victims speak: Part I. An empirical review of the empirical literature, 1981–2001. *Psychiatry: Interpersonal and Biological Processes, 65,* 207–239. http://dx.doi.org/ 10.1521/psyc.65.3.207.20173.

Noullet, C., Lating, J. M., Kirkhart, M. W., Dewey, R., & Everly, G. S., Jr. (2018). Effects of pastoral crisis intervention training on resilience and compassion fatigue in clergy: A pilot study. *Spirituality in Clinical Practice, 5*, 1–7. http://dx.doi.org/10.1037/scp0000158.

Parad, H. J. (1971). Crisis intervention. In R. Morris (Ed.), *Encyclopedia of social work* (Vol. 1, pp. 196–202). New York, NY: National Association of Social Workers.

Parad, L. G., & Parad, H. J. (1968a). A study of crisis-oriented planned short-term treatment: Part I. *Social Casework, 49*, 346–355. http://dx.doi.org/10.1177/104438946804900603.

Parad, L. G., & Parad, H. J. (1968b). A study of crisis-oriented planned short-term treatment: Part II. Social Casework, 49, 418–426. http://dx.doi.org/10.1177/104438946804900705.

Raphael, B. (1986). *When disaster strikes: How individuals and communities cope with catastrophe*. New York, NY: Basic Books.

Rapoport, L. (1965) The state of crisis: Some theoretical considerations. In H. Parad (Ed.), *Crisis intervention: Selected readings* (pp. 22–31). New York, NY: Family Service Association of America.

Reinert, M., Nguyen, T. & Fritze, D. (2021). *The state of mental health in America*. Alexandria, VA: Mental Health America. https://mhanational .org/research-reports/2021-state-mental-health-america.

Stapleton, A. B., Lating, J. M., Kirkhart, M., & Everly, G. S., Jr. (2006). Effects of medical crisis intervention on anxiety, depression, and posttraumatic stress symptoms: A meta-analysis. *Psychiatric Quarterly, 77*, 231–238. http://dx.doi.org/10.1007/s11126-006-9010-2.

United Nations (2020). *Policy brief: COVID-19 and the need for action on mental health*. Geneva, Switzerland: United Nations. https://www.un.org /sites/un2.un.org/files/un_policy_brief-covid_and_mental_health _final.pdf.

US Census Bureau (2021, February). *Week 24 household pulse survey: February 3–February 15*. https://www.census.gov/data/tables/2021/demo /hhp/hhp24.html.

World Health Organization. (2018). *mhGAP operations manual: Mental Health Gap Action Programme (mhGAP)*. Geneva, Switzerland: World Health Organization.

THIRTEEN | Self Care

Taking Care of Others Begins (and Ends)
with Taking Care of Yourself

The Need For Self-Care

We cannot relieve the suffering of others if we,
ourselves, are suffering.

—HAWES CLEVER

So, you've completed the Johns Hopkins RAPID PFA model intervention. If all goes well, you deserve to reflect, if not bask, fondly on a job well done. You were present, you developed rapport through empathy and reflective listening, you assessed thoroughly, you prioritized the relevance of the signs and symptoms you heard, you provided successful cognitive and stress management interventions, and you ended by leaving the person in a very good emotional place with referral and contact information if needed. You were the consummate helper.

What about you? Even if all goes well, and even if you're successful in the majority of your future interventions, listening to others tell their traumatic experiences can take an emotional toll on you over time. No matter how well-intentioned you are, and no matter how resilient you envision yourself to be, repeated exposure to traumatic events, even if it's only for short periods of time, can adversely affect you. You can't help at times but absorb some of the sadness, picture the stories, and be affected by the hardship that you hear. You are not immune.

It is important to be aware of some of the negative emotional reactions a psychological first aid (PFA) provider might experience while working with individuals following critical incidents. Some of the terms that describe these consequences include *vicarious traumatization, secondary traumatic stress* (STS), *burnout,* and *compassion fatigue.* The constructs of vicarious traumatization, STS, and compassion fatigue are often used interchangeably, but they are actually considered distinct conditions (Rothschild & Rand, 2006). Because you might hear these different terms during your work as a crisis interventionist, we briefly define and differentiate each of them here. Various risk factors that increase the potential of experiencing some of these adverse effects are also provided. To help mitigate their impact, we describe the construct of self-care and offer ways to develop, foster, and engage in this important protective mechanism.

Terminology
Vicarious Traumatization

Vicarious traumatization refers generally to the process of *cognitive changes in beliefs* (e.g., changes in sense of self or changes in one's worldview about issues of safety, trust, control, and spiritual beliefs) that occurs from continual interactions with trauma survivors (Pearlman & McCann, 1995). These cumulative experiences can have deleterious effects on those who provide care and require ways for providers to mitigate their impact.

Secondary Traumatic Stress

Secondary traumatic stress, which emphasizes *behavioral symptoms* one experiences as compared to intrinsic cognitive changes that are the hallmark of vicarious traumatization, may result from creating an empathic relationship with an individual who is suffering from exposure to trauma and then being exposed to the intense experiences of that person (Figley, 1983, 1995; Figley & Kleber, 1995). Secondary traumatic stress has been described as a compilation of symptoms in the helper that include reliving aspects of the distressing story or traumatic event, avoiding reminders of this event or story, and experiencing psychosocial and physiological symptoms, such as heightened irritability, sleep disturbances, quick temper, sadness, withdrawal, and task avoidance (Figley, 2002). In essence, "the primary exposure to traumatic events by one person becomes the traumatizing event for the second person" (Harrison & Westwood, 2009, p. 204), and the symptoms of STS mirror the symptoms of posttraumatic stress disorder (PTSD; see chapter 3).

Burnout

PFA providers must also be aware of burnout. Herbert Freudenberger (1984), who coined the term, described burnout as "a depletion or exhaustion of a person's mental and physical resources attributed to his or her prolonged, yet unsuccessful striving toward unrealistic expectations, internally or externally derived" (p. 223). Burnout is considered to be more than fatigue and overwork, and it is not related specifically to working with individuals who have experienced traumatic events. It's *mental and physical exhaustion*. Typically, burnout builds up over time, evidenced by emotional exhaustion, loss of empathy, reduced satisfaction with work, and other signs of personal distress, such as insomnia, irritability, relationship difficulties, and increased substance use (Freudenberger, 1975; Maslach & Jackson, 1981). These symptoms and signs are often seen in disorders such as depression, generalized anxiety disorder, and substance use (see chapter 3).

Compassion Fatigue

Compassion fatigue might best be defined as a syndrome that consists of a combination of symptoms from secondary traumatic stress and burnout (Adams, Boscarino, & Figley, 2006; Bride, Radney, & Figley, 2007; Newell, & MacNeil, 2010). Compassion fatigue generally describes the *aggregate experience of emotional and physical fatigue* that a helper can experience as a result of the protracted use of empathy expended when exposed to another person's actual or anticipated emotions when discussing distressing stories or events (Benoit, McCarthy, & LeRoy, 2007; Figley, 2002; Rothschild & Rand, 2006). The term *compassion fatigue* was originally coined by Joinson (1992) in a nursing magazine to describe the condition of nurses who were exhausted from their daily care of patients in the emergency room. Similar to burnout, compassion fatigue is thought to be a cumulative process that develops over time, whereas vicarious trauma and secondary traumatic stress onset often occur more immediately (Newell & MacNeil, 2010).

Compassion fatigue captures the essence of what might happen to a PFA provider who spends considerable time providing the RAPID model. However, there might be occasions in which there are physical or emotional triggers, such as the physical resemblance of a victim to a family member or the victim being a child that is close to your child's age that elicit unexpected yet ardent responses from you in an isolated interaction that might be more consistent with STS. Regardless of which construct you consider, it is important to note some of the signs and symptoms that can occur. Not surprisingly, many of these elements parallel the signs of distress noted previously in this text, as well as symptoms of PTSD, depression, anxiety, and substance use noted in chapter 3. While recognizing and appreciating this overlap, we nonetheless offer the following considerations for someone who might be experiencing the effects of compassion fatigue:

- Feelings of emotional depletion or exhaustion
- Neglecting physical, emotional, and spiritual needs
- Diminished quiet time to reflect and replenish oneself
- Feeling unappreciated
- Diminished ability to be empathetic
- Decreased sense of purpose and accomplishment
- Decreased concentration
- Reduced satisfaction and fulfillment in doing PFA
- Providing diminished quality of PFA
- Irritability

- Fatigue
- Insomnia
- Cynicism
- Increased substance abuse
- Relationship difficulties (Carter & Barnett, 2014; McCarthy & Frieze, 1999; Wicks, Parsons, & Capps, 2003)

Risk Factors

No one is immune from the potential emotional consequences of providing PFA. Moreover, having some of the signs and symptoms is not a sign of personal weakness. No different than the sound advice you give as a PFA provider to normalize others' reactions in the aftermath of a traumatic event, keep in mind that the reactions you might be experiencing as a result of a traumatic encounter are likely related to the event, not an inherent personality weakness on your part. You are experiencing what might be considered normal reactions to exposure to particularly abnormal events.

However, certain potential risk factors might exacerbate the chances of adverse emotional impact. For example, there is thought to be a dose-response relation regarding exposure, which means that the more times you are asked to provide PFA, the greater the likelihood of compassion fatigue. Also, events that involve children, are human-made (as compared to natural disasters), affect people whom you know, and involve a greater number of casualties all pose inherent risks of increasing symptoms in providers, such as compassion fatigue (Neria, Nandi, & Galea, 2008).

It is important to know yourself. Everyone is different. We all have unique personality styles formed from an amalgam of genetics (nature) and social learning (nurture). This combination might influence why you have chosen to help others, your eagerness to respond to critical incidents, your assertiveness in volunteering to approach others who are in apparent need, and even your choice of profession. This combination also might influence the kind of events and the type of person who "gets to you," and this might be evidenced by how you respond to someone who is demanding, aggressive, angry, physically imposing, or exceedingly emotional. Know what affects you personally or what is likely to affect you. In other words be aware of your "stuff" or your blind spots. At a more extreme level, it has been noted that providers with preexisting anxiety, mood disorders, or trauma history (particularly child abuse), while usually very adept at evidencing empathy, tend over time to be at a higher risk for possible detrimental outcomes, such as compassion fatigue (Dunkley & Whelan, 2006; Nelson-Gardell & Harris, 2003).

Individuals, agencies, and organizations need to acknowledge the existence of constructs such as compassion fatigue as a distinct, dynamic, and unintended liability in working with those who have experienced a traumatic event. In addition, individuals and organizations need to have preventative measures and other self-care strategies to try and help avert compassion fatigue from occurring or to mitigate its impact. In a study of 125 responders to Hurricanes Katrina and Rita who completed standardized measures, including a self-care assessment, it was found that providers who engaged in self-care practices during their response had higher levels of compassion satisfaction (deriving satisfaction from their work) than those who practiced fewer self-care strategies (Lambert & Lawson, 2013). Given the current, pervasive impact of COVID-19, there are recommendations for all of us, with a particular emphasis on frontline workers, to engage in self-care strategies (Centers for Disease Control and Prevention, 2020; Cullen, Gulati, & Kelly, 2020).

Self-care

Self-care is considered an ongoing, if not lifelong, process that entails self-awareness and self-regulation in balancing psychological, physical, and spiritual needs that enhance our connection with our self and others (Baker, 2003). The essence of self-care is to promote wellness and effective functioning. It is intended to be infused within a productive lifestyle, so it is not meant to be an added burden or obligation that one "needs" to do (Carter & Barnett, 2014). Naturally, what constitutes self-care varies from person to person, but there are certain general aspects and practices of self-care for PFA providers that should be considered.

Organizational Practices

Once you are trained to provide PFA, you become part of a large family of other PFA providers, who, not surprisingly, are typically accomplished, eager helpers. One of the best ways to practice preventative self-care as a PFA provider is to develop and foster consultative, supervisory, or more personal mentoring relationships with those who are seasoned PFA providers. This can occur at either an organizational or individual level. If these providers exist within your organization, then they are clearly easier to find. During field service, you might consider developing a buddy system wherein a mutual agreement is made to monitor and foster one another's psychological well-being. However, if you are not part of an organization that supports and offers PFA, you can possibly locate providers who are willing to serve as consultants or provide mutual aid through organizations such as the International Critical Incident Stress Foundation (ICISF.org) or the Green Cross.

A primary way to use these consultants is through activities referred to as postaction staff support (PASS) (Potter & LaBerteaux, 2000). PASS enables PFA providers to discuss with other, often more experienced, PFA providers some of the following:

1. How successful was the PFA provider in implementing the procedural steps of the RAPID protocol. That is, did the provider follow the steps and meet the expected criteria described in each of the steps?

2. How successful was the PFA provider in navigating the person in possible distress through the emotional domains associated with the RAPID model? That is, did the provider help the person to discuss a traumatic event from a cognitive framework to a more affective or emotional framework and then return back to a more cognitive level of functioning?

3. What was the emotional impact of the intervention on the PFA provider? That is, did the intervention resonate with the provider,

did it strike a personal, emotional chord? How is the provider doing emotionally?

PASS is used more frequently when the PFA provider is a novice in implementing the RAPID model and is then most effectively used on an as-need basis when the PFA provider is experienced. However, regardless of how seasoned a PFA provider becomes, PASS should continue to be used to foster self-care and to counter professional isolation or to check in with a colleague to process the emotional impact of PFA work. Anecdotal data exists of seasoned crisis interventionists, driving home after successful interventions, realizing that tears were streaming down their face. No one is immune.

Although reaching out to colleagues can help effectively facilitate self-care needs, the bulk of self-care involves attending to one's own personal needs. As noted, self-care should be considered and infused as part of your daily lifestyle. However, it is especially important not to dismiss these strategies if you are providing crisis intervention services on a prolonged basis. But regardless of the duration of the response or the frequency of responding, self-care should be considered. A traumatic event is considered a toxin that enters the body and the mind. We adhere to the notion that good information is one of the most effective antidotes to the toxin. Therefore, included here, where appropriate, is relevant information related to why one should implement certain self-care strategies. However, let us be clear in the statement of our bias on this topic. We strongly believe that *any* organization engaged in emergency and disaster response has an ethical obligation to provide some form of organized psychological support to its responders. The most widely used model of integrated, multicomponent support for responders is critical incident stress management (CISM). Everly and Mitchell (2016) provide a useful practitioner's guide to the implementation of CISM programs.

Basic Self-Care Behavioral Elements

Self-care often starts with attending to the most basic physiological needs, such as maintaining adequate amounts of sleep, nutrition, and exercise (Norcross & Guy, 2007). These basic physiological needs were covered in chapter 8 as part of intervention suggestions you would most often give to others. However, are you adhering to them? Are you getting seven to nine hours of sleep per night, and eating a balanced diet, if at times you're eating at all during an initial response to an ongoing critical incident? One of the first activities to jettison when we are under consider stress is exercise. Are you maintaining an exercise routine that entails 30 or more minutes or moderate-intensity exercise five days a week or 20 minutes of vigorous-intensity activity three days a week? Hey, if it's important enough for others, it has to be important enough for you.

Spiritual/Religious Self-Care

Another relevant consideration addressed in chapters 8 and 11 is the incorporation of faith or spiritual care into one's self-care. Data generally support the role of spiritual and religious beliefs in positively influencing one's physical and emotional health and overall well-being (Van der Merwe, Van Eeden, & Van Deventer, 2010). Whereas spirituality generally refers to one's personal connection with realities larger than oneself, religion in essence formalizes and organizes through rituals or behaviors what the spiritual individual might be experiencing (Josephson & Peteet, 2004). As Richards and Bergin (1997, p. 13) note, "It is possible to be religious without being spiritual and spiritual without being religious." Wicks (2006) refers to our spiritual life as also our "interior" or "inner" life and suggests that it "includes those psychological and spiritual factors that provide us with inner strength, a sound attitude, and a sense of honesty or transparency" (p. 88).

It has been demonstrated that individuals who use religious coping strategies (e.g., seeking spiritual support) have more stress-related growth (i.e., potential to develop positive outcomes, such as broadened perspectives and deepened relationships, following traumatic events) and higher self-esteem (Ano & Vasconcelles, 2005; Yakushko, 2005). Moreover, and particularly relevant for this text, those who are intrinsically religious (i.e., who use religion as an end in and of itself as compared to using religion as a means of achieving some other end) have been noted to have higher distress shortly after a traumatic event but lower severity of PTSD symptoms over time, as well as increased posttraumatic growth eight months or more after the trauma (Schaefer, Blazer, & Koenig, 2008). Also, in a qualitative study assessing how therapists help protect themselves from the risks of vicarious traumatization, they acknowledged that a spiritual interconnection renewed their conviction in people's resilience, their ability to grow in the wake of trauma, that life is about more than suffering, that their efforts in helping are meaningful, and that they are not solely responsible in their efforts to help others try and heal (Harrison & Westwood, 2009). Therefore, the incorporation of spiritual and religious beliefs or, more broadly, infusing a spiritual connection into self-care practices might lead to an enhanced meaning and purpose in life and a better and more unconditional acceptance and compassion for others (Ellis, 2000).

Other Self-Care Strategies

Self-care is a personal endeavor that will likely change over time. The suggestions that follow are not meant to be prescriptive or exhaustive. The important caveat to remember is that self-care is meant to be an enjoyable way to remove you from the pressures, challenges, and burdens of not only responding to a critical incident but also of reacting to the daily stresses associated with your personal and professional life. Practicing self-care is not meant to be an additional obligation or another source of stress in your life. It is meant to create a balance. With this in mind, consider some of the following, much of which will enhance behavioral or spiritual well-being:

- Take a quiet, relaxing walk.
- Write in a journal. (In fact, and as depicted in the scenario, there are data to suggest that writing about emotional topics is cathartic and provides long-term improvement in mood, behavior changes, and physical functioning [Pennebaker, 1999].)
- Listen to music.
- Find opportunities to laugh.

- Take a bath instead of a quick shower.
- Connect with a friend via telephone or e-mail.
- Cultivate a hobby.
- Spend time outdoors.
- Play with your children.
- Develop a practice of mindfulness (being present in the moment).
- Implement and practice other relaxation strategies. (As noted in chapter 8, effective relaxation strategies can include meditation or active and passive neuromuscular relaxation. For a description of these, including step-by-step instructions, see Everly & Lating, 2019.)
- Make plans to get away from work to spend time with family or friends.
- Be proactive in making plans with others.
- Take your vacation time.
- Manage your time better to schedule interruptions and breaks.
- Take time for reflection.
- Sleep in when you can.
- Maintain clear personal and professional boundaries (i.e., say no when it's simply too much).

The overall goal of a crisis interventionist is to remain empathically connected, present, and engaged while being balanced and protected from the adverse effects of providing PFA. There are many who consider their role in providing PFA as a privilege and purpose in helping others. We agree. However, in an effort to enhance your longevity in this calling, it is prudent, if not relevant, to take care of yourself.

Developing a Plan

That which is not planned does not get done. So be sure to make a plan for self-care (see Everly and Lating [2019] for a compendium of stress management tactics). Consider using the following structure for prolonged service in the field (although these basic principles can be useful on short call-outs for service in the field as well):

1. Preactivation/Deployment
    a. Establish a reliable means of communicating with family/ friends, coworkers, supervisors.
    b. Identify transportation resources to and from the work site.
    c. If possible, anticipate and prepare for the situation in which you will be working.
        i. What will be the physical challenges?
        ii. What will be the psychological challenges?
        iii. Will there be any cultural or communication challenges (see chapter 11)?
        iv. What will be the policy and means for referring those who need custodial care?
2. During Field Service
    a. Identify transportation resources.
    b. Identify any organizational or local resources for staff support, daily as well as extraordinary.
    c. Can you create a buddy system?
    d. Monitor your daily stress levels.
    e. Identify resources for stress management (e.g., spiritual, physical exercise, hobbies).
    f. Communicate with friends/family back home.
    g. Stay informed on hometown news.
    h. Keep a daily journal.
    i. Establish routines, especially someone to eat breakfast or dinner with on a regular basis.
3. After Field Service (Transitioning Back Home)
    a. Use PASS.
    b. Informally communicate your experiences.
    c. Use stress management techniques.
    d. Write a "lessons learned" summary of your experience.

KEY POINT SUMMARY

1. PFA providers must recognize a possible emotional toll associated with exposure to those who have experienced critical incidents.

2. *Emotional toll* has been referred to by various terms, including *vicarious traumatization, secondary traumatic stress (STS), burnout,* and *compassion fatigue.*

3. The term *compassion fatigue,* which is considered a combination of STS and burnout, seems to fit what might happen to a PFA provider if she provides services over time. However, its important to be familiar with possible signs and symptoms regardless of what term is used to denote this emotional exposure.

4. Duration, frequency, and type of exposure are risk factors that increase the chances for adverse emotional impact.

5. The construct of self-care is a lifelong process to help balance psychological, physical, and spiritual needs.

6. Organizational self-care strategies can include postaction staff support, and personal self-care should include such strategies as sleeping, eating, exercising, and spiritual care.

7. Developing a plan, among the other suggestions, is the best way to enhance self-care.

References

Adams, R. E., Boscarino, J. A., & Figley, C. R. (2006). Compassion fatigue and psychological distress among social workers: A validation study. *American Journal of Orthopsychiatry, 76,* 103–108. http://dx.doi.org/10.1037/0002-9432.76.1.103.

Ano, G. G., & Vasconcelles, E. B. (2005). Religious coping and psychological adjustment to stress: A meta-analysis. *Journal of Clinical Psychology, 61,* 461–480. http://dx.doi.org/10.1002/jclp.20049.

Baker, E. K. (2003). *Caring for ourselves: A therapist's guide to personal and professional well-being.* Washington, DC: American Psychological Association.

Benoit, L. G., McCarthy, P., & LeRoy, B. S. (2007). When you care enough to do your very best: Genetic counselor experiences of compassion fatigue. *Journal of Genetic Counseling, 16,* 299–312. http://dx.doi.org/10.1007/s10897-006-9072-1.

Bride, B. E., Radney, M., & Figley, C. R. (2007). Measuring compassion fatigue. *Clinical Social Work Journal, 35,* 155–163. http://dx.doi.org/10.1007/S10615 -007-0091-7.

Carter, L. A., & Barnett, J. E. (2014). *Self-care for clinicians in training: A guide to psychological wellness for graduate students in training.* New York, NY: Oxford University Press.

Centers for Disease Control and Prevention (2020). *COVID-19: Stress and coping.* Retrieved August 26, 2021 from https://www.cdc.gov/coronavirus /2019-ncov/daily-life-coping/stress-coping/index.html.

Cullen, W., Gulati, G., & Kelly, B. D. (2020). Mental health in the COVID-19 pandemic. *QJM: An International Journal of Medicine, 113,* 311–312. http://dx .doi.org/10.1093/qjmed/hcaa110.

Dunkley, J., & Whelan, T. A. (2006). Vicarious traumatization: Current status and future directions. *British Journal of Guidance and Counseling, 34,* 107–116. http://dx.doi.org/10.1080/03069880500483166.

Ellis, A. (2000). Spiritual goals and spirited values in psychotherapy. *Journal of Individual Psychology, 56,* 277–284.

Everly, G. S., Jr., & Lating, J. M. (2019). *A clinical guide to the treatment of the human stress response* (4th ed.). New York, NY: Springer Nature.

Everly, G. S., Jr., & Mitchell, J. T. (2016). *Critical Incident Stress Management (CISM): A practitioner's review of CISM.* Ellicott City, MD: International Critical Incident Stress Foundation.

Figley, C. R. (1983). Catastrophes: An overview of family reactions. In C. R. Figley & H. I. McCubbin (Eds.), *Stress and the family: Vol. 2; Coping with catastrophe* (pp. 3–20). New York, NY: Brunner/Mazel.

Figley, C. R. (1995). *Compassion fatigue: Coping with secondary traumatic stress disorder in those who treat the traumatized.* Levittown, PA: Brunner/Mazel.

Figley, C. R. (2002). Compassion fatigue: Psychotherapists' chronic lack of self-care. *Journal of Clinical Psychology, 58,* 1433–1441. http://dx.doi.org/10 .1002/jclp.10090.

Figley, C. R., & Kleber, R. J. (1995). Beyond the "victim": Secondary traumatic stress. In R. J. Kleber, C. R. Figley, & B. P. R. Gersons (Eds.), *Beyond trauma: Cultural and societal dynamics* (pp. 75–98). New York, NY: Plenum.

Freudenberger, H. J. (1975). The staff burn-out syndrome in alternative institutions. *Professional Psychology: Research and Practice, 12,* 73–82. http://dx.doi.org/10.1037/h0086411.

Freudenberger, H. J. (1984). Impaired clinicians: Coping with burnout. In P. A. Keller & L. Ritt (Eds.), *Innovations in clinical practice: A sourcebook* (Vol. 3, pp. 221–228). Sarasota, FL: Professional Resource Exchange.

Harrison, R. L., & Westwood, M. J. (2009). Preventing vicarious traumatization of mental health therapists: Identifying protective practices. *Psychotherapy Theory, Research, Practice, Training, 46*, 203–219. http://dx.doi.org/10.1037/a0016081.

Joinson, C. (1992). Coping with compassion fatigue. *Nursing, 22*, 116–122.

Josephson, A. M., & Peteet, J. R. (Eds.). (2004). *Handbook of spirituality and worldview in clinical practice.* Arlington, VA: American Psychiatric Publishing.

Lambert, S. F., & Lawson, G. (2013). Resilience of professional counselors following Hurricanes Katrina and Rita. *Journal of Counseling and Development, 91*, 261–268. http://dx.doi.org/10.1002/j.1556-6676.2013.00094.x.

Maslach, C., & Jackson, S. E. (1981). The measurement of experienced burnout. *Journal of Occupational Behaviour, 2*, 99–113. http://dx.doi.org/10.1002/job.4030020205.

McCarthy, W. C., & Frieze, I. H. (1999). Negative aspects of therapy: Client perceptions of therapists' social influence, burnout, and quality of care. *Journal of Social Issues, 55*, 33–50. http://dx.doi.org/10.1111/0022-4537.00103.

Nelson-Gardell, D., & Harris, D. (2003). Childhood abuse history, secondary traumatic stress, and child welfare workers. *Child Welfare, 82*, 5–26.

Neria, Y., Nandi, A., & Galea, S. (2008). Post-traumatic stress disorder following disasters: A systematic review. *Psychological Medicine, 38*, 467–480. http://dx.doi.org/10.1017/S0033291707001353.

Newell, J. M., & MacNeil, G. (2010). Professional burnout, vicarious trauma, secondary traumatic stress, and compassion fatigue: A review of theoretical terms, risk factors, and preventative methods for clinicians and researchers. *Best Practices in Mental Health, 6*, 57–67.

Norcross, J. C., & Guy, J. D. (2007). *Leaving it at the office: A guide to psychotherapist self-care.* New York, NY: Guilford Press.

Pearlman, L. A., & McCann, P. S. (1995). Vicarious traumatization: An empirical study of the effects of trauma work on trauma therapists. *Journal of Psychology: Research and Practice, 26*, 558–565. http://dx.doi.org/10.1037/0735-7028.26.6.558.

Pennebaker, J. W. (1999). The effects of traumatic disclosure on physical and mental health: The values of writing and talking about upsetting events. *International Journal of Emergency Mental Health, 1*, 9–18.

Potter, D., & LaBerteaux, P. (2000). Debriefing the debriefers: Operational guidelines. In G. S. Everly, Jr., & J. T. Mitchell (Eds.), *Critical incident stress management: Advanced group crisis interventions a workbook* (pp. 111–113). Ellicott City, MD: International Critical Incident Stress Foundation.

Richards, P. S., & Bergin, A. E. (1997). *A spiritual strategy for counseling and psychotherapy.* Washington, DC: American Psychological Association.

Rothschild, B., & Rand, M. (2006). *Help for the helper, self-care strategies for managing burnout and stress: The psychophysiology of compassion fatigue and vicarious trauma.* New York, NY: W. W. Norton.

Schaefer, F. C., Blazer, D. G., & Koenig, H. G. (2008). Religious and spiritual factors and the consequences of trauma: A review and model of the interrelationship. *International Journal of Psychiatry in Medicine, 38,* 507–524. http://dx.doi.org/10.2190/PM.38.4.i.

Van der Merwe, E. K., Van Eeden, C., & Van Deventer, H. J. M. (2010). A psychological perspective on god-belief as a course of well-being and meaning. *HTS Teologiese Studies / Theological Studies, 66,* 1–10.

Wicks, R. J. (2006). *Overcoming secondary stress in medical and nursing practice: A guide to professional resilience and personal well-being.* New York, NY: Oxford University Press.

Wicks, R. J., Parsons, R., & Capps, D. (2003). *Clinical handbook of pastoral counseling* (Vol. 3). Mahwah, NJ: Paulist Press.

Yakushko, O. (2005). Influence of social support, existential well-being, and stress over sexual orientation on self-esteem of gay, lesbian, and bisexual individuals. *International Journal for the Advancement of Counseling, 27,* 131–143. http://dx.doi.org/10.1007/s10447-005-2259-6.

APPENDIX

A Breathing Technique

THE USE OF DIAPHRAGMATIC BREATHING can be helpful in promoting a more relaxed state and can be taught during the intervention stage of the RAPID PFA model. The following is a technique developed by G. S. Everly, Jr., that has been shown to induce rapidly (within 30 to 60 seconds) a state of relaxation. Start with the description as if instructing a patient before moving on to the steps.

> When we find ourselves in anxiety-producing situations, our heart rates increase, our stomachs may become upset, and our thoughts may race uncontrollably. It is during such episodes that we require fast-acting relief. The brief exercise described below has been found effective in reducing most of the stress reactions that we suffer from during acute exposures to stressors—it is, in effect, a quick way to "calm down" in the face of a stressful situation.

> Step 1. Assume a comfortable position. Rest your left hand (palm down) on top of your abdomen, over your navel. Now place your right hand so that it rests comfortably on your left. Your eyes can remain open. However, it is usually easier to complete Step 2 with your eyes closed.

Step 2.   Imagine a hollow bottle, or pouch, lying internally beneath the point at which your hands are resting. Begin to inhale. As you inhale imagine that the air is entering through your nose and descending to fill that internal pouch. Your hands will rise as you fill the pouch with air. As you continue to inhale, imagine the pouch being filled to the top. Your rib cage and upper chest will continue the wavelike rise that was begun at your navel. The total length of your inhalation should be two seconds for the first week or two, then possibly lengthening to two and a half or three seconds as you progress in skill development.

Step 3.   Hold your breath. Keep the air inside the pouch. Repeat to yourself the phrase, "My body is calm." This step should last no more than two seconds.

Step 4.   Slowly begin to exhale—to empty the pouch. As you do, repeat to yourself the phrase, "My body is quiet." As you exhale, you will feel your raised abdomen and chest recede. This step should last as long as the two preceding steps, or may last one second longer, after a week or two of practice. (*Note.* Step 1 need only be used during the first week or so, as you learn to breathe deeply. Once you master that skill, you may omit that step.) Only repeat this four-step exercise three to five times in succession. Should you begin to feel light-headed, stop at that point. If light-headedness recurs with continued practice, simply shorten the length of the inhalation and/or decrease the number of times you repeat the exercise in succession.

Make this exercise a ritual in the morning, afternoon, and evening, as well as during stressful situations. Because this form of relaxation is a skill, practice it at least 10 to 20 times a day. At first you may not notice any on-the-spot relaxation. However, after a week or two of regular practice, you will increase your capabilities to relax temporarily. Remember, you need to *practice regularly* if you are going to master this skill. Regular, consistent practice . . . will ultimately lead to the development of a more calm and relaxed attitude—a sort of anti-stress attitude—and when you do have stressful moments, they will be far less severe.

Reprinted with permission from G. S. Everly, Jr., and J. M. Lating, *A Clinical Guide to the Treatment of the Human Stress Response*, 4th ed. (New York, NY: Springer, 2019).

INDEX

Page numbers in *italics* refer to illustrations.

About the Authors

George S. Everly, Jr., PhD, ABPP, FAPA, FAPM, is acknowledged as a pioneer in the fields of psychological trauma and disaster mental health. He is an award-winning author and researcher. Dr. Everly holds appointments as professor in the Center for Humanitarian Health in the Johns Hopkins Bloomberg School of Public Health and associate professor (part time) in psychiatry and behavioral sciences at the Johns Hopkins School of Medicine. He was formerly professor of psychology at Loyola University in Maryland (core faculty) and a member of the Johns Hopkins Center for Public Health Preparedness. In addition, he has served on the adjunct faculties of the Federal Emergency Management Agency (FEMA) and the FBI's National Academy at Quantico, Virginia. Dr. Everly holds honorary professorships at the Universidad de Flores, Buenos Aires, Argentina, and Universidad de Weiner, Lima, Peru. He was a member of the Centers for Disease Control and Prevention Mental Health Collaboration Committee (having chaired the mental health competency development subcommittee), the Infrastructure Expert Team within the US Department of Homeland Security, and the National Voluntary Organizations Active in Disaster (NVOAD) Emotional & Spiritual Care Committee, as well as the NVOAD Early Psychological Intervention subcommittee. He has been an advisor to the Hospital Authority of Hong Kong. Dr. Everly is cofounder of and serves as a nongovernmental representative to the United Nations (UN) for the International Critical Incident Stress Foundation, a nonprofit UN-affiliated public health and safety organization. He was formerly Distinguished Visiting Professor, Universidad de Flores (Argentina) and senior research advisor in the Social Development Office, Office of His Highness, the Amir of Kuwait, State of Kuwait. Before these appointments, Dr. Everly was a Harvard Scholar, visiting in psychology, Harvard University; a visiting lecturer in medicine, Harvard Medical School; and chief psychologist and director of behavioral medicine for Johns Hopkins Homewood Hospital Center.

Dr. Everly is a fellow of the American Psychological Association and a fellow of the American Institute of Stress. In addition, he has been awarded the Fellow's Medal of the Academy of Consultation and Liaison Psychiatry and the Professor's Medal of the Universidad de Weiner (Peru). He is the author, coauthor, or editor of 20 textbooks and more than 100 professional papers. Dr. Everly has received numerous awards, including the Director's Award from the Bureau of Alcohol, Tobacco, Firearms, and Explosives; the World Trade Center Response Award from the New York Police Department; the Certificate of Honor from the Baltimore Police Department; the Honor Award from the American Red Cross; the Leadership Award from the American Red Cross; and the Maryland Psychological Association's Award for Scientific Contributions to Psychology. Dr. Everly was the recipient of the University of Maryland's College of Health and Human Performance's 50th Anniversary Outstanding Alumni Award and was recognized as a Pioneer in Clinical Traumatology by the Traumatology Institute of Florida State University. He was awarded the Susan Hamilton Award for consensus building and collaboration in disaster mental health. He served as the mental health chairperson for the Central Maryland Chapter of the American Red Cross, where he was cofounder of the disaster mental health network. In addition, he assisted in the development of the state of Maryland Disaster Mental Health Corps and Maryland's Disaster Spiritual Care Corps. Dr. Everly was the 39th president of the Maryland Psychological Association. He has given invited lectures in 25 countries on six continents. His works have been translated into Russian, Arabic, Swedish, Polish, Portuguese, Japanese, Chinese, German, Korean, and Spanish.

Jeffrey M. Lating, PhD, earned his BA in psychology from Swarthmore College in 1985 and his PhD in clinical psychology in 1991 from the University of Georgia. He also completed a postdoctoral fellowship in medical psychology at the Johns Hopkins Hospital in 1993. He was the director of clinical training at the Union Memorial Hospital in Baltimore from 1993 to 1996, and the chief psychologist there from 1996 to 1998. He is currently a professor of psychology at Loyola University Maryland and was the director of clinical training of the doctoral program in clinical psychology at Loyola from 2000 to 2013. Dr. Lating is also a faculty member of the International Critical Incident Stress Foundation. From 2005 to 2009, he served on the Maryland State Board of Examiners of Psychologists. He has coedited and coauthored six books in the areas of stress and posttraumatic stress.

Dr. Lating has also served as a clinical consultant and crisis-management trainer with FEMA; the Federal Bureau of Alcohol, Tobacco, Firearms and Explosives (ATF); the Association of Professional Flight Attendants (APFA); the United States Senate Employee Assistant Program; the US Department of State; the US Department of Labor; the United Steelworkers (USW); the Danish Military; the Edmonton Police Service; the Royal Canadian Mounted Police (RCMP); the Swiss Air Navigation Services; and the World Bank. He also consulted and provided clinical interventions and training with the US Secret Service's Employee Assistance Program in New York City in the days after the terrorist attacks of September 11, 2001.